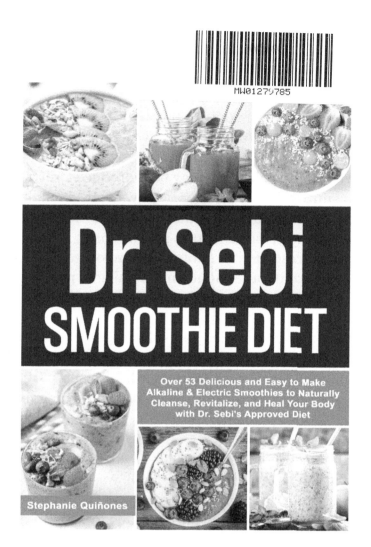

Dr. Sebi Smoothie Diet:
Over 53 Delicious and Easy to Make Alkaline & Electric Smoothies to Naturally Cleanse, Revitalize, and Heal Your Body with Dr. Sebi's Approved Diet

Ebook ASIN: ASIN: B08LH5FB1B
ISBN: 9798550345450

Dedication

I would like to dedicate this book to Dr. Sebi for sharing the knowledge of the power of Alkaline, Electric Food, and the Medicinal Herbs diet that heals the body and cures diseases. You have inspired me to change my nutrition in my life and make life so much satisfying to live.

I honored your hardwork and determination in providing us with the knowledge to overcome adversity. I will not take this for granted and will pass along your powerful knowledge about health and nutrition through the Alkaline and Electric Foods diet.

Table Of Content

Introduction

Alfredo Darrington Bowman, fondly called Dr. Sebi, was a healer and herbalist who practiced in the United States in the 20th century and 21st century. Some of his works and principles remain through even in these modern times. Dr. Sebi was born in 1933 in Honduras and is an African. As he grew older, he became dissatisfied with some of the Western medical practices and began looking for new solutions to some of the serious medical conditions of the 20th century. After visiting a herbalist in Mexico who healed him of his asthma, diabetes, and impotence, he went back to Honduras. He began his healing practice, and after years of research, he developed a treatment called the African Bioelectric Cell Food Therapy, which he claimed could cure a wide range of illnesses, including AIDS, which was one of the major medical conditions of the 20th century. After developing his treatment, Bowman established his center in Honduras and began to sell his products to the United States. He eventually moved to New York, where he met a lot of legal opposition as a result of his claims, and after a while, he moved to California.

Dr. Sebi's diet was based on the use of natural foods and vegetables to revitalize the body's cells and internal cleansing. Dr. Sebi believed that eating certain foods and staying away from some would help the body to detoxify and achieve an alkaline state, thereby reducing the risk of diseases. He also believed that acidity in the body was one of the major causes of disease infection. While a lot of people criticized his beliefs and practices because they did not have any scientific backing and did not follow any of the medical principles of that time, some subscribed to his beliefs, and he soon began to develop a clientele such as Lisa Lopes, Steven Seagal, Eddie Murphy, John Travolta, and Michael Jackson. In August 2016, Alfredo Bowman died on the way to the hospital as a result of some complications. His teachings and treatment methods have spread across the world after his death, with more people making use of it than ever before.

CHAPTER 1

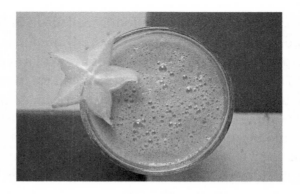

UNDERSTANDING THE MEANING OF ALKALINE

How to properly use this book?

In this book, I have outlined principles that can guide readers to a better and healthy living. These shouldn't only be seen as a diet, instead it should be seen as a healthy eating lifestyle. Therefore to apply these principles outlined in this book, these are the things to do:

- Strictly follow Dr. Sebi's nutritional diet guide.
- Ensure you consume only foods that fall under the electric foods category
- Avoid acidic-based foods and only consume alkaline-based foods
- Consume great tea, instead of coffee
- Several tips and life hacks have been highlighted in the book to aid your smoothie lifestyle
- Learn how-to and prepare smoothies as strictly outlined in this book.
- A list of medicinal plants have been given in the book, ensure you explore their medical advantages

In conclusion, the principles in this book are not just outlined for diet purposes; these principles are outlined so that you can make them a part or a whole in your healthy eating lifestyle.

When we hear the word 'Alkaline,' we immediately think about alkaline water that we have heard so much about the litmus paper that we used for experiments in high school. While those do give us an understanding of what alkaline is no matter how little. Alkaline refers to the pH level of a substance, whether it is food, water, the human body. Alkaline also refers to the dissolution of a solution called alkali (derived from the Arabic word 'qali,' which means from the ashes'). An alkali does not have to be a particular substance or material, and it can even be food or water. In fact, the stomach releases an alkaline liquid called bile that AIDS in the digestion of food, and the mixture of the bile with the food and other enzymes in the stomach creates an alkaline solution. Apart from the stomach, the small intestine also has enzymes that work at a pH of 12. Alkaline solutions can be formed through natural processes like erosion and can also be manufactured in a laboratory. Since it is basic, alkaline solutions are used in laboratories to make chemical reactions neutral or basic. It is these alkaline solutions that turn red litmus paper blue as we were shown in high school. Like acid, the level of alkaline in a particular food or substance is measured using pH levels (a pH level helps to determine how acidic or alkaline a substance is). However, determining the strength of an alkaline material requires a little more than pH levels, and this is where a little chemistry comes in. To determine the strength of alkaline, you have to add a universal indicator (a universal indicator is a combination of other indicators e.g., methyl blue) to your substance but when it comes to food or water, all you need to know most times are their pH levels especially if you are on a diet. Before I continue, I must mention that any substance with a pH level greater than 7 is alkaline, while a substance with a pH level of 7 is neutral.

Now that we have gotten that out of the way, how does an alkaline diet work? Am I going to have to work out and give up a lot of the food I love for this diet? An alkaline diet starts with a promise; a promise that by the end of the diet, you would achieve not only your dream body but also rid your body of all the toxins and acids that made your body that way in the first place and by the time you are done, your body will have a fresh start. An alkaline diet is a diet that aims to increase the body's alkalinity and make it less acidic. This diet recommends complete departure from foods such as sugar, processed foods, snacks, dairy products, red meat, and other food items that can increase the body's acidity. This diet majorly focuses on the use of fruits and vegetables to maintain a healthy weight while ridding the body of harmful toxins and acids that had caused unhealthy weight gain. The premise of this diet is that it can alter your body's pH levels in a way that would be beneficial to it by eating certain foods that have high levels of alkaline. Proponents of this diet also claim that following this diet can help to reduce the risk of cancer, kidney stones, diabetes and can also help to improve health and overall wellness. The alkaline diet is about bringing back good old-fashioned healthy eating habits where natural foods were placed above sugars, dairy, and processed food. When it comes to cancer, some studies suggest that cancer thrives in an acidic environment; therefore, when you increase your body's alkalinity, you are reducing your body's risk of having cancer. However, there is still a lot of debate on how an alkaline diet helps to prevent cancer, but one sure thing is that an alkaline diet does aid in losing weight and improving the body's overall function. When starting the alkaline diet, you need to have it at the back of your mind that you would be giving up about 90% of the foods you are used to, and you cannot just order take-outs any time you like during the diet.

You cannot eat any of the dairy products you are used to eating or the chocolates that you adore so much. If you are an early morning coffee type of person, know that you would not be allowed to take coffee or any form of caffeine during the diet, and alcohol is also prohibited during the diet. This diet does a complete reset of the body and restores it to its healthy fat-burning state. Nuts and seeds are also allowed in this diet since they increase alkalinity in the body. Since you are not going to be buying any processed or canned goods during this diet, you would have to cook and prep most of your meals and drinks if you do not want to drink water. Also, there would be little or no need to exercise since your body would be running on a lesser amount of calories than it used to have. This diet is completely vegetarian due to the absence of meat, and it is also gluten-free, so make sure that anything you buy at the grocery store is gluten-free. This diet also reduces the risk of allergies since many of the foods we eat that would result in allergies are cut out as well and, you can do this diet on your own because it is easy to follow, and there are hardly any complications when following this diet.

Importance of pH in the Body

Have you heard of the term 'pH balance' and wondered what it meant? There are acids in our body which are necessary for digestion and other bodily functions and, there is alkaline in the body as well. The body has its way of maintaining pH balance, but sometimes, it might not be able to as a result of the foods and drinks that we take. Most of the foods we eat are acidic, and consuming them in large quantities can cause an imbalance, which would not be good for you and your health. Our cells live and die, and maintaining the body's alkalinity helps the cells to stay alive and function. When our bodies get too acidic, it prevents oxygen from getting to the cells, which can result in the body storing fat in the cells and can lead to the growth of more fat cells, which is the last thing that our bodies need.

If there is no pH balance in the body or if it is too acidic, it could lead to the lungs or kidney malfunctioning, plus, the imbalance could lead to serious medical conditions like acidosis and alkalosis that require medical treatment and not just changes in diet. Maintaining pH balance or a little more alkalinity, allows your body to remain the way it is, and does not put any strain on it whatsoever. Too much acidity or pH imbalance would spell bad news for your immune system as the imbalance would cause your immune system to weaken gradually, thereby making your body more susceptible to diseases. Also, you would begin to feel more fatigued, stressed out, and more prone to mood swings because your body uses essential alkaline nutrients from different parts of the body to make up for what is missing. As a result of the lack of energy you would be experiencing, it would be hard for you to go through the day and carry out all your activities without some form of supplement to keep you going. Like your nervous system, your muscles and joints would also suffer from the pH imbalance. As the acid starts to build up, it would begin to accumulate in your joints and damage your cartilages (the damage done to your cartilages could lead to severe medical conditions such as arthritis). Hyperacidity (the presence of high acid levels in the body) could lead to pimples, blemishes, and other breakouts on the skin because your pH level is imbalanced. Also, the skin could gradually grow weaker and become more susceptible to damage and premature aging.

However, as much as too much acidity is bad, too much alkalinity in the body is dangerous as well, but this rarely happens compared to cases of hyperacidity.

Health Consequences of Acidity in the Body

Acidosis is a health condition that occurs as a result of too much acid on the body fluids, and it occurs when the kidney and the lungs cannot maintain the body's pH balance. When the lungs fail to expel enough CO_2 from the body as a result of conditions like asthma, obesity, chest muscle weakness, chest injuries, alcohol overuse, and the likes, it results in a buildup of CO_2 which increases the body's acidity and the same applies to the kidney. If the kidneys cannot expel enough acid or remove too much alkaline from the body, it would also result in an acid buildup. Apart from the lungs and kidneys, other factors like obesity, dehydration, diabetes, methanol poisoning, aspirin, a high-fat diet, and kidney failure could also cause acidosis. Most symptoms and health consequences of acidosis are popular and can easily be mistaken for something else, but if your body is going through acidosis, you will experience:

- Drowsiness
- Confusion
- Sleepiness
- Headaches that you cannot trace to anything you had done during the day
- Lack of appetite
- Jaundice

- Increase in heart rate since your body is working overtime to make up for the imbalance and;
- A breath that smells a little bit like fruits

These are not all the symptoms, but if you are experiencing any one of the symptoms or most of them at the same time, make sure to go and see a medical professional before things get out of hand. As I mentioned earlier, any food or substance with a pH level that is less than 7 is acidic and for you to maintain your body's pH levels, you can either avoid these foods completely or limit your consumption of them especially when you are not on a diet and just want to maintain a healthy lifestyle. For any food to be considered acidic, it must have a pH level of 4 or lower, and some of these foods that tend to cause more acidity in the body include:

- Sugar
- Grains such as wheat
- Some dairy products such as cheese, full cream milk, ice cream and butter
- Processed foods
- Fish
- Red meat and processed meats like turkey and canned beef
- Soda and sweetened beverages
- Supplements and foods that are high in protein
- Foods that have a high-fat content

Generally, a lot of citrus fruits are acidic in nature and can contribute to the level of acidity in the body. When drinking fruit juice, especially those that are acidic, make sure to keep them away from your teeth as they can cause decay when consumed too much. On a normal day, these fruits, drinks, and foods are okay as long as they are not consumed regularly and do not aggravate any underlying medical condition. A lot of vegetables, especially fresh vegetables, are not acidic, but for your alkaline diet, make sure to avoid sauerkraut as it is acidic in nature. Another thing to note is that most of the fruits mentioned are only acidic in nature, and when metabolized by the body along with other alkaline ingredients, they can serve as blood alkalizing agents.

Fresh or Frozen Food, Does it Matter?

Foods are embedded with nutrients – vitamins, fibers, antioxidants and minerals. Therefore freezing is a very safe way to protect and increase the nutritional life of foods. However, people wrongly believe that frozen foods are much less nutritious than fresh foods. There still seems to be a huge controversy about the healthiness of frozen foods. Therefore, this section of the book is dedicated to give answers to the controversies. I will attempt to give answers to whether to go for frozen foods or fresh foods and when.

To start with, it is important to state that the season in which we find ourselves dictates what we can choose – either fresh foods or frozen food. For instance, during winter, fresh foods are limited, scarce and expensive; hence many of us are forced to approach frozen or canned foods. This is so because frozen foods are the cheaper and better option during the winter season. More so, two recent independent studies found that in 66 percent of cases, frozen fruit and vegetables contained more antioxidants such as vitamin C, polyphenols, beta carotene and lutein compared to fresh varieties stored in the fridge for three days. Not only do antioxidants help keep our immune system healthy, but studies suggest they also help fight illnesses such as heart disease and cancer. Note however that, whether your food is fresh or frozen, it is important to know that how you cook your food, fresh or frozen, is vital to retaining the nutrients. As there are some vitamins that are sensitive to heat or leach out into water. Steaming, stir-frying or microwaving vegetables means little water is used and food is cooked for a short period of time. By adhering to this procedure, you can ensure that your fresh or frozen foods retain more nutrients than if they're boiled for a long time. At this juncture, it is important to note that some frozen foods are healthier than others. Therefore, in order to identify a healthy frozen meal from an unhealthy one, you need to closely observe the nutrition label. Examine the number of calories, sodium, saturated fat, and sugar per serving. Some nutritional experts recommend frozen meals contain less than 600 mg of sodium, a maximum of 25 grams of fat, and total calories around 400. Look at the ingredient list, too.

Ingredients will be listed from largest to smallest in quantity, so pay most attention to the first few items you see. That said, if you see any foreign food names towards the end of the list, this usually means it's a preservative or additive.

More Than Just Fresh Fruits and Vegetable

Broccoli: Frozen broccoli had higher levels of vitamin C and lutein and four times more beta carotene (fresh had more polyphenols).

Carrots: Frozen carrots contained three times more lutein, twice as much beta carotene and more vitamin C and polyphenols than fresh.

Blueberries: Frozen had more vitamin C, polyphenols and anthocyanins (fresh contained more lutein and beta carotene).

Peas and Sweet Corn: No significant difference between frozen and fresh.

What are Classifications of Foods?

The food we consume daily plays a vital role in determining who and what we are. It also goes a long way in ensuring that we live longer than our parents who knew not the understanding of food classes or balanced diets. Hence, it is crucial to eat healthy foods. In the world today, there are numerous dishes, and you may be stumped on the foods to combine to achieve a balanced diet. This is why Classifying food became important.

Classification of food simply means the subdivision of food into various groups, and globally, there are seven recognized classes of food, namely:

1. Carbohydrates
2. Proteins
3. Fats
4. Minerals
5. Vitamins

6. Fibers
7. Water

Note that the classification of foods is dependent on two types of nutrients; they are:

- **Macronutrients:**

    These nutrients are needed majorly by the body for the effective functions of various organs. They are responsible for preserving energy, and they are necessary at all times. Examples of food classes under this type of nutrients are Carbohydrates, Proteins, Fats, Fibers, and Water.

- **Micronutrients:**

    These nutrients are needed in smaller amounts in the body, and they majorly consist of vitamins and minerals.

    Note that macro and micronutrients are the difference between healthy and sick. Thus, when one or both are insufficient in the body, the body deteriorates, allowing the easy entry of harmful diseases.

    Here's a broader view of the classes of food and their importance to bodily health.

- **Carbohydrates:**

    Generally, Carbohydrates are often referred to as energy-giving foods. They provide the body with the required energy for its daily activities. Examples of Carbohydrates include wheat, barley, flour, maize, rice, and all other starchy foods and grains.

Carbohydrates are subdivided into three different groups, namely:

1. **Polysaccharides:** This type of carbohydrates is tough to digest, the hardest of all saccharides.

2. **Disaccharides:** This is formed using two Monosaccharides, and a good example is sucrose.

3. **Monosaccharides:** This is basic Carbohydrates, the simplest form of Carbohydrates.

Finally, albeit taking Carbohydrates is good for energy generation, excess consumption could lead to numerous health issues such as diabetes and other heart diseases.

- **Proteins**

These are also referred to as body-building foods. They are vital in cell growth, muscle development, and general improvement of metabolism. Examples of foods in this class include fish, chicken, dairy products, beans, etc.

You should know that there are two subtypes of protein used by the body. First, the non-essential protein generated by our body itself and a shortage of it would cause little or no harm to the body. While the second, the essential protein, is necessary because it determines the lifespan of all animals, humans inclusive. These essential Proteins are majorly found in dairy products, meats, fish, eggs, etc.

- **Fats**

Fats are also known as energy-giving foods. They are used to maintain energy balance, aid the regulation of body temperature and the intake of vitamins into the body. Examples of fats include nuts, avocados, fish, soya beans, butter, olive oil, and so on.

There are two types of fat, namely:

1. **Saturated Fats:** Saturated fats Includes butter, cheese, processed meat, and other cookies. Although these fats have their health benefits, excessive

consumption of foods with high saturated fat isn't advised to prevent a spike in cholesterol levels and reduce the chances of heart diseases.

2. **Unsaturated Fats:** Unsaturated Fats include fats from fruits and nuts, fishes rich in omega-3, and various plant generated oils.

Medical experts advised that people consume food rich in unsaturated fats because it helps reduce cholesterol levels.

- **Minerals**

Minerals are a type of Micronutrients not needed in large quantities in the body. They are elements vital to the longevity of one's life. They include calcium, magnesium, zinc, iron, and so on.

Minerals are necessary to keep the body at optimal health. They are equally responsible for muscle development, the durability of bones and teeth, etc.

Lastly, minerals can be found in numerous kinds of foods, veggies, and fruits.

- **Vitamins**

Vitamins are another class of food not required in large quantities. They improve brain health and boost our immune system. Examples of vitamins include Folic acid, Thiamine, Riboflavin, and so on.

Finally, note that Vitamins can be found in fruits and almost every food in the world.

- **Fibers**

Fibers aid digestion. Once they are included in one's diet, they cannot be absorbed by the body due to the absence of enzymes. Generally, they are a subtype of Carbohydrates, which consists of cellulose. Examples of Fibers include broccoli, oranges, beans, green bean, lentils, cereals, onions, currants, corn, etc.

They are vital to the smooth run of our digestive system by keeping all cholesterol levels in check. Fibers are also used as preventive diets for diseases such as diabetes, CAD coronary artillery disease, cancer, and so on.

- **Water**

We all know water as that colorless and odorless substance that we can't live without. However, do you know that water constitutes a significant part of humans? I bet you don't!

The good news is water can be found in every food available to man. Yet, it is still compulsory to take some liters of water daily for easy digestion and to stay hydrated.

While this class of food is simply a mixture of hydrogen and oxygen to get H2O, however, it is still crucial to achieving a balanced diet.

Conclusively, just like the old saying goes, *"don't dig your grave with your knife and fork."* hence, it is crucial to know the classification of foods. Also, knowing it is not enough, but living by it and eating food that won't stress the body, foods that aren't detrimental to your health, foods that aren't acidic is vital to longevity and ensure that we live a life free of various health troubles. This is why plant-based nutrition is advised. Learn to be creative with your diet and ensure that your classes of food are balanced. This way, you won't be killing yourself with your fork and knife, and there will be a greater chance that you'll live longer than your folks.

Why Smoothies are an Easier Path to a Healthier You

Smoothies have been part of cleanses, diets, and have even become a part of many people's daily lives. It is more than just a combination of fruits and vegetables as their health benefits are too many to count. You can make anything into a smoothie and that is why it is regarded as one of the healthiest items you can add to your diet. Here are some benefits of adding smoothie to your diet.

- **Added Nutrients:** Food items like nuts, yoghurt, leafy vegetables, and of course fruits, can be added to smoothies which means that you can get all the nutrients that your body needs from just one sip. There are different types of smoothies ranging from green smoothies to fruit smoothies, and protein smoothies and based on their composition, all of them have the nutrients your body needs to function on a daily basis. They contain protein, fats, antioxidants, vitamins, and minerals which means that smoothies are basically a meal on their own. These nutrients helps to build your immunity, maintain bodily functions, aid digestion, and flush out toxins from your body

- **Supports Weight Loss:** Smoothies have long been hailed as one of the secrets to weight loss due to the fact that you can replace at least a meal or two per day with a glass of smoothie. If your smoothie is homemade with fats and proteins, it helps to keep you fuller for longer which allows your body to tap into the fat reserve available in the body and boost metabolism. Since they keep you fuller for longer and have a little bit of natural sugars in them, it can also help to curb cravings thereby reducing the amount of junk food a person eats per day meaning that the total calories consumed per day, will most likely be cut in half.

- **It Helps to Prevent Dehydration:** As we go through the day, it is easy to get dehydrated without even knowing it since most of us tend to go without water for most of the day and not even notice it. The only time it would be brought to our attention is through the feeling of tiredness, dizziness or fatigue and then, we might not still be aware that our body is severely dehydrated. Smoothies are light and can be carried around anywhere you go and since water is one of the components in a smoothie, you will stay hydrated throughout the day while getting the energy you need to go through the day without slowing down. Do you know that dehydration can cause your skin to look dull? Being dehydrated for long periods of the day can make your skin look dull, dry and itchy but half of that problem can easily be solved by drinking more water per day as well as taking some nutrients that helps the skin regenerate all of which can be provided by smoothies.

- **Cleanses the Body:** If you are looking for a way to clear your body of all the toxins, then a smoothie diet is the way to go. The body has a natural way of cleansing the body of toxins but a little boost will help the process go faster. Based on its composition, smoothies are filled with a lot of nutrients that the body needs to function and by going on a smoothie diet, you are cutting out some of the foods that led to the buildup of the toxins in the body which gives your body time to flush them out effectively.

- **Controls Cravings:** smoothies are renowned for the immense nutrients and flavor. Due to the presence of a lot of protein and other nutrients, consumers of smoothie can subdue food cravings and stay away from consuming junk foods.

- **Enhances the Body's Immunity:** when we talk about, we are referring to your body's ability to fight against diseases, bacteria and/pathogens. When you consume smoothies made of ingredients that contain nutrients like beta-carotene, you enhance/boost your body's immune system.

- **Aids Fight Against Sleep Disorder:** people around the world belonging to diverse age groups often experience problems relating to sleep disorder, insomnia and restlessness. A healthy glass of smoothie made up of bananas, kiwi and oats provides the body with magnesium and calcium in a good amount. A sufficient amount of calcium and magnesium in the body will induce sleep and help the body maintain a healthy sleeping pattern.

- **Provides Liquid Food Benefits:** nutrition and health experts all over the world suggest that consuming liquid foods aids better digestion. Smoothies contain blended fruits and vegetables in liquid form; hence it is easy for the body to break down.

- **Accelerated Brain Power:** it is no news that certain fruits and vegetables contribute to brain power and mental alertness. More so, mental alertness and brain power is greatly increased and boosted by fruits and vegetables which are rich in omega-3 fatty. When you consume smoothies containing ingredients rich in omega-3 fatty, you are consuming smoothies that can heal your brain work faster.

- **Improves Bone and Tooth Health:** a regular intake of calcium, vitamin D3 and vitamin K are nutrients that aid the improvement of bone and tooth health. Smoothies that contain spinach, green vegetables and citrus fruits as chief ingredients are a great source of these nutrients.

- **Keeps Blood Sugar in Check:** diabetes and high blood sugar are the commonest diseases that bother humans around the world today. People who have imbalanced sugar levels in their blood are prone to several complications. Therefore, having a smoothie rich in nutrients but low in calories can reduce or completely eradicate this imbalance sugar level in your body. Smoothies containing fresh fruits and vegetables are a great choice to supply nutrients to the body without increasing your sugar level.

- **Reduces Chances of Having Cancer:** several studies and reports all over the world have published research showing that foods like cabbage, broccoli, and cauliflower are helpful in fighting against cancer. Smoothies that attack cancer-growing factors prove very helpful in preventing cancer. Also, fruits like blueberries, strawberries and grapes are rich in antioxidants which preclude the growth of carcinogens.

- **Balances Hormonal Functioning:** hormones play a large role in regulating our day-to-day functions. However, any imbalance in hormonal levels can lead to huge repercussions. More so, hormonal imbalances can make the body susceptible to several health hazards. Therefore, to keep your hormones working properly, all you need is a refreshing glass of smoothie.

- **Smoothies are Better Alternatives for Juices:** when it comes to health benefits, smoothies are a better alternative for juices. Juices often lack the pulp of fruits and vegetables, while smoothies consist of every part of fruits and vegetables.

CHAPTER 2

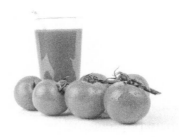

THE AMAZING HEALTH BENEFITS OF THE ALKALINE SMOOTHIE DIET

Since the alkaline diet was introduced, many studies and research have been carried out to validate its benefits. In this chapter, we will be discussing those benefits and some of the scientific research backing them up.

Like most diets, the alkaline smoothie diet also aims to prevent weight gain and promote weight loss. Since most of what you will be consuming are fruits and vegetables, that means that you would be consuming fewer calories than you are used to; also, the diet is low in fat and sugar, which makes it one of the best weight loss solutions. If you want to take the alkaline smoothie without going on a diet, it can also help you lose weight as long as you combine it with exercise and a healthy lifestyle. Another benefit of this diet is that it helps to improve kidney health. According to a study conducted in 2017, most people's typical diet is usually acidic, which can pose a challenge to the health of your kidneys. A lower acid diet can prevent or reduce the risk of kidney disease, and for those who already have the disease, the alkaline diet can help slow it down.

Heart disease is one of the leading causes of death worldwide because a lot of people have poor nutrition, unhealthy lifestyles, and do not do as much exercise or activity as they need to. The alkaline diet can help raise the levels of growth hormone, which helps lower the risk of heart disease also since the diet is low in fat, sugars, and calories help to lower or prevent the risk of heart disease. This diet also eliminates red and processed meat from the causes of heart disease since red meat is not consumed during the diet. Alkaline smoothie diet can also help relieve or lessen back pain (however, it is uncertain whether or not alkaline smoothies help with chronic pain). Osteoporosis is one of the major causes of bone fractures in elderly people and females. The alkaline smoothie diet reduces the amount of calcium that is lost in the urine, which helps to lower the risk of osteoporosis. The smoothie diet is filled with fruits and vegetables, which helps to promote bone health.

As people grow older, they tend to lose muscle mass, which increases the risk of a person falling and having fractures. The alkaline diet helps to promote muscle health by increasing muscle mass, especially among females. Cancer cells thrive in an acidic environment, and since you will be consuming fruits and vegetables that promote pH balance and alkalinity in the body, it can help to reduce the risk of cancer. If you are not on a diet, having a glass of alkaline smoothie a day along with exercise and a healthy lifestyle can also help to reduce the risk of having cancer.

Best Alkaline Food

Alkaline foods are important as they help to bring balance to your body and provide it with a lot of nutrients. Generally, you should be consuming around 60% of alkaline foods and 40% of acidic foods to maintain the body's pH balance. Indulging yourself in excess snacks, sugars, and red meat is not good for your health, and if you are willing to make a change, here are some foods that would be an excellent addition to your diet.

- **Green Leafy Vegetables:** Most of the leafy vegetables around serve as alkaline agents and would be an excellent addition to any diet. Also, they provide essential nutrients that the body needs to carry out its daily functions, and some of the greens you can add to your diet include spinach, lettuce, kale, Swiss chard, celery, parsley, mustard greens, and arugula.

- **Broccoli and cauliflower:** Broccoli and cauliflower not only provide phytochemicals that are needed by the body, but they are also excellent sources of alkaline to your diet or eating plan. Mix the broccoli and cauliflower with other vegetables like beans, green peas, and capsicum, and you would have all the alkaline and nutrients that your body needs in just one bite.

- **Tomatoes:** When uncooked, tomatoes are an excellent alkaline source and still provide a good amount of alkaline to the body even when cooked. They also provide nutrients like Vitamin C, Vitamin B6, and some digestive enzymes to the body. Add some tomatoes to your morning omelets or eat some slices as a snack with a little bit of pink sea salt for some additional flavor.

- **Almonds:** Almonds are great alkaline snacks during a diet and are also an excellent addition to any recipe. The high magnesium content in almonds makes it alkaline-forming, and the healthy fats that are found in almonds make them nutritious and filling. On your alkaline smoothie diet, almonds can be added to the smoothie if you do not mind the texture that it would bring.

- **Garlic:** Garlic is anti-inflammatory and a good source of alkaline, making it one of the best foods you can add to your diet. It has also been proven to help prevent some diseases, improve the immune system, and fight against bacteria in the body.

- **Avocado:** Avocado is one of the superfoods that nature provided as it is packed with nutrients and all sorts of deliciousness. Avocados contain healthy fat, which is good for the body and helps prevent weight gain. Apart from being an alkalizing agent, avocado also helps to improve heart health, and it is anti-inflammatory.

- **Red Onion:** Onions are a good source of Vitamin C and have been proven to have anti-bacterial and anti-inflammatory effects. Cooking it lightly with a bit of healthy fat helps to improve its alkalinity, but it also provides a lot of nutritional benefits when eaten raw.

- **Sea salt and seaweed:** Sea salt and seaweed contain ten times more nutrients than any other vegetable grown on land, which makes it an amazing addition to any diet since they provide a lot of nutrients to any meal. They are also good sources of alkaline and seaweed can be used to make certain dishes while the sea salt can be used to spice up meals such as omelets, salads, soups, and the likes

- **Seasonal fruits:** Any dietitian or nutritionist would tell you that adding seasonal fruits to your diet is extremely beneficial to your health. Seasonal fruits are filled with vitamins, minerals, and antioxidants, which means they provide nutrients that are essential to different parts of the body; also, they are excellent sources of alkaline. Examples of seasonal fruits include kiwi, pineapple, persimmon, watermelon, grapefruit, apricots, apples, and nectarine.

- **Nuts:** Do you like munching on nuts when hunger starts to kick in? Well, it turns out you have been moving in the right direction as nuts are a good source of healthy fat and alkaline. Since they are high in calories, they should not be eaten all the time, and when eaten, it should be in small quantities. Nuts like cashew nuts and chestnuts should be included in your diet plan.

Hybrid Foods

Hybrid foods are the products of the combination of two similar types of fruits. Is it okay to include these hybrid foods in a diet? Do these hybrid fruits and vegetables provide the body with as many nutrients as normal fruits and vegetables? Some people have raised the argument that all fruits and vegetables are hybrid technically due to pollination and other factors; however, that does not mean that hybrid fruits and vegetables are as good as the ones available. Most hybrid fruits are man-made and products of the laboratory. Hybrid foods contain three times the amount of sugar and might not contain as many nutrients as non-hybrid foods so, eating hybrid foods might give your body some problems as it is not used to such high amounts of sugar and mineral imbalance in a fruit or vegetable. Since most of these hybrid foods are grown in the labs and need special conditions to grow, it might contain harmful and toxic chemicals that would not be good for your body. Your overall health and wellbeing depend on your awareness of these hybrid foods and how they can affect your health. When on a diet, it is best to stay away from them and stick to the fruits that you know since the nutrients and health benefits to be gotten from them are guaranteed.

Why are Hybrid and Man-made Foods Dangerous for Your Health?

Today around the world, we have been inundated with hybrid or hybridized foods, whether you agree with me or not. If you are observant, you would have seen a watermelon shaped like a basketball rather than the conventional oblong shaped watermelon. Well, the basketball shaped watermelon is a man-made/hybrid fruit. As much as these hybrid foods are described by food engineers as "convenient and easy," they actually do more harm to us than good. Hybrid, as well as, mad-made foods are dangerous and harmful for so many reasons.

First, hybrid foods do not possess vital electrics. What do I mean by this? Hybrid foods lack vital mineral vital content. Hybrid foods are unnaturally lacking in sugar and completely off in mineral and compound ratio. When we consume a lot of hybrid food, our body doesn't get the necessary mineral it needs. More so, the sugar produced by hybrid foods is not entirely recognized by the liver and pancreas. Hybrid foods are commonly attacked by different forms of fungi and are much more susceptible to decay. Commercially produced hybrid crops are not immune enough to withstand diseases, infestation, and other natural factors like fungus or infections. The corn that was hybridized for the first time in 1930 also died due to less capability to withstand harsh conditions and resist pests.

Now let's talk about hybrid seeds. They are quite expensive to procure and it is practically impossible to save them to grow another generation of plants. In fact, some of these plants will grow fruit that is seedless, meaning that there is no way to save the seeds and produce another generation. Hence, you will need to buy hybrid seeds again the next year in order to grow your garden. Let's even assume that you plant hybrid seeds, and that the fruit does end up having seeds. I hate to break it to you that the next generation of plants grown from these new seeds is not guaranteed to be anything like the last generation. In fact, the next generation of plants may be less vigorous, less productive, or more susceptible to disease than the previous generation. Even worse, the next generation might not be able to produce fruit at all. Worst case scenario, the seeds will not germinate, and you won't get any plants at all.

More so, when a hybrid seed is produced that has some desired characteristic, it often comes at the expense of another good trait. For example, seeds that grow into plants with larger fruit may also have fruit that is less tasty. Perhaps this is because the fruit contains more water, so the plant cannot produce fruit that tastes quite as good as the smaller ones. I have often found this to be the case with oranges – in my view, the smaller oranges often have much more intense flavour than the large ones. In addition to having more water, larger fruits may also have lower nutrient content. The reason is that the plant has been bred to produce larger fruit, without necessarily acquiring the ability to absorb more nutrients from the soil. This means that the plant cannot provide enough nutrients to give the fruit the same nutritional value (pound for pound) as smaller fruit. The same problem could stem from increased yields: if a plant produces twice as much fruit, but takes up the same amount of nutrients, then every fruit may have half the nutrients of a normal one.

Awesome and Nutritious Ingredients to Add to Your Smoothie

Smoothies are the best cool, creamy, delicious meal-in-a-glass. Before you finally blend your smoothie ingredients, below are some nutritious/awesome ingredients you can add to your smoothie:

- **Dark, Leafy Greens:** greens are awesome additions for smoothies. However, don't be afraid to try out beet roots, celery (with leaves) or other dark, leafy greens. Greens are low in sugars and calories, and provide more iron and protein than fruit. They're also bursting with fibre, folate, and phytonutrients like carotenoids, saponins and flavonoids. All greens help support a healthy weight, keep bowel movements regular, fight inflammation and decrease the risk of chronic disease. If you have a difficult time consuming greens, adding them to smoothies are a great way to increase your intake.

- **Nuts, Nut Butters and Seeds:** Veggies are vital in a smoothie, but protein will stabilize your blood sugars and keep you feeling full. Peanut butter, other nut butters, nuts and seeds provide protein — and they also provide heart-healthy fat. Choose natural peanut or almond butter (all peanuts or almonds, no fillers), or add walnut halves to boost your omega-3 intake. As much these nuts, nut butters, and flax seeds are nutrient-filled – they also contain a high level of calories, so you need to be mindful of the portion sizes.

- **Cruciferous Vegetables:** examples of cruciferous vegetables are: shredded cabbage, leafy green kale, Bok Choy, etc. Cruciferous vegetables are nutrient-rich gems containing glucosinolates. These glucosinolates are an anti-inflammatory phytonutrient. More so, cruciferous vegetables when added to your smoothie is another way for you to increase your overall vegetable consumption.

- **Dairy products:** dairy products such as Greek yogurt, milk and other milk alternatives are another great source of protein, which can help make your smoothie a true meal replacement that keeps you away from hunger or crazy unwanted junks cravings. These dairy products are a great alternative as a source for protein instead of protein powders, which often come with unwanted flavours and sugar. If you want to add any of these dairy products to your smoothie, I highly recommend that you use non-fat, plain Greek yogurt, unflavoured almond milk or soy milk.

- **Berries:** if you desire a lot of fruits in your smoothie, then this one's for you. Berries such as raspberries, blueberries, strawberries and other berries add a sweet and tart flavour to your smoothie. More so, these berries are rich in fibre which helps you stay full. Berries, according to research, also contain antioxidants which are suggested to cancer-fighting properties. It is also important to state that, berries are low on glycaemic index; therefore, berries won't spike your blood sugar as quickly as other fruits would. So instead of using ice cubes for your smoothies, frozen bags of mixed berries is a nutritious alternative.

Tips to Lose Weight with Ease

All body sizes are beautiful but it is completely okay if you want to shed a few pounds. People lose weight for a variety of reasons and as easy as it is to decide to lose weight, losing weight isn't the easiest thing in the world to do. However, here are a few tips that will make your journey easier and melt everything away with ease.

- **Intermittent Fasting:** As someone who is serious about making their weight loss journey a success, I am sure that you might have heard of intermittent fasting.

Intermittent fasting is basically about setting certain periods of the day for eating and not about what to eat. It doesn't regulate the type of food you can take only the time you can eat. There are different options when it comes to intermittent fasting such as 12:12, 14:10, 16:8, 20:4, OMAD, and many more so, you can start small then choose a different option when you are ready. By putting a time restraint on meals, intermittent fasting gives the body time to digest the meals that have been eating as well as tap into its reserve. When doing this fast, restrain from eating foods that would sabotage it.

- **Take Protein, Healthy Fats, and Water:** Protein and fats helps to keep the body fuller for longer which helps to reduce the calories you consume each day. Sometimes we mistake dehydration for hunger so always keep a bottle of water beside you so that when you feel hungry, you can really decide if your body really needs food or just water.

- **Move Around All the Time:** For some exercising is not an option but that doesn't mean you have to sit around all day. Rather than driving around, you can take a walk especially if where you are going to is a place you can easily walk to. Move around as frequently as you can. To help, you can get a smartwatch that would help calculate the number of steps you take per day and you have to make sure that you remain consistent.

- **Look for Healthier Alternatives:** Nowadays, there are a lot of healthier options to some of the foods we cannot live without. If you cannot remove snacks completely from your diet, then look for healthy snacks that you can take that won't hinder your progress.

- **Get a Lot of Sleep:** Do not compromise on getting 8 hours of sleep every day and do not change your sleeping pattern all of a sudden, Stick to it for as long as you can and if you want to change your pattern, then do it slowly so that your body can adjust to it.

- **Go on a Diet You Can Turn into a Lifestyle:** Majority of us workout or go on diets solely for the purpose of losing weight but once we get the results, we go back to our old ways and gain the weight back. Before you go on a diet or start a workout regime, ensure it is something that you can add to your life and do on a regular basis so that you can lose the weight and keep it off completely.

- **Drink Water, Especially Before Meals:** it is often said that drinking water can aid weight loss – and that's true. Drinking water can aid metabolism by over 20%, thereby helping you burn a few calories. Recent studies have also shown that drinking 17 ounces of water about half an hour before meals helped dieters eat fewer calories and lose over 40% more weight than those who didn't drink water.

- **Drink Green Tea:** green tea has many benefits, one of them being weight loss. Besides containing a small amount of caffeine, green tea also contains a powerful antioxidant called catechins, which are believed to possess properties that work with caffeine to aid fat burning.

- **Reduce Added Sugar:** added sugar is one of the worst ingredients in the 21st century modern diet. Sadly, some people consume way too much added sugar. Recent researches have shown that excessive consumption of sugar will result in obesity, type 2 diabetes and heart disease. If you are serious about losing weight, then you need to cut back on added sugar.

- **Do Aerobic Exercise and Lift Weights:** doing aerobic exercises and lifting weights is an excellent way to burn calories and improves your physical and mental health. Aerobic exercise is particularly known for aiding the loss of belly fat, and the unhealthy fat that tend to build up around your organs.

- **Avoid Sugary Drinks, Including Soda and Fruit Juice:** we already know excessive sugar is bad, but sugar in liquid form is even worse. Recent studies have also shown that the calories from liquid sugar is one of the most fattening aspects of the 21st century diet. Consume a lot of fruits, but limit or avoid fruit juice altogether. If you are serious about losing weight, then you need to stay away from all forms of liquid sugar.

- **Don't Diet, Eat Healthily:** dieting isn't such a bad idea, however they are rarely effective in the long run. If anything, people who diet tend to gain more weight over time. More so, studies have even shown that dieting is a consistent predictor of future weight gain. So, instead of going on a diet, aim to eat healthily and focus on nourishing your body appropriately instead of depriving it. When you eat healthily and nourish your body appropriately, weight loss should then follow naturally.

- **Consume More Fiber:** fiber is often recommended for weight loss. Studies have shown fiber can increase satiety and help you control your weight over the long run.

To see results, make sure you remain consistent. 70 percent of weight loss has to do with diet so make sure you watch what you eat and get enough sleep so that you can see the best results. To maintain the results, make this into a lifestyle.

Use Smoothies as a Meal Replacement or Snack

Smoothies these days are more than just drinks that you slurp in between meals or on the way to work. With a few additions, they can replace meals without you noticing the difference and can also serve as healthy snacks. The composition of smoothies depends on what you need it to do.

The smoothie you take as a quick snack in the morning is completely different from the one you need in the afternoon to keep you going for the rest of the day. For you to consider your smoothie a meal, you need to include a lot of heavy ingredients that would satisfy you as much as a regular meal would. You would have to include proteins such as Greek yoghurt, chia seeds, nuts, and nut butter, a little bit of fiber which you can get from oats, and pumpkins, and you definitely need some healthy fat like avocado, coconut oil, and flax seeds in your smoothie. All these ingredients when blended together with some fruits and vegetables, will give you the fullness you get from eating a regular meal.

While smoothies as a meal needs to be a little on the heavy side, as a snack you do not need to worry about adding these heavy ingredients. All you need is fruits and vegetables in the right portions, then a little bit of water or you can also add some Greek yoghurt or peanut butter if you want a little added flavor in your smoothie. If you are preparing it yourself, you can also throw in a few chia seeds for the added protein.

When going on a smoothie diet, it is best to make it at home so that you can be certain that the ingredients would be beneficial to you and help further your goals. Most store-bought smoothies are packed with sugars and it might not be easy for you to determine its composition which might hinder your progress. Remember to buy enough products to last at least a week and change some ingredients so that the process can remain fun for you.

CHAPTER 3

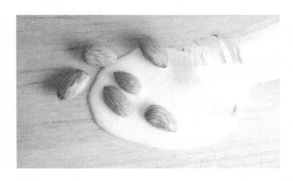

DELICIOUS ALKALINE SMOOTHIES

With all the information you need on the alkaline diet at your fingertips, it is time to go into it properly. In this chapter, we will discuss some smoothies that would be great for your diet and help you start your day feeling refreshed with a good pH. These smoothies are also great for people with acid reflux or indigestion because it contains no acid. Remember that once you start the diet, you could be cutting away up to 90% of what you are used to consuming, but it would be worth it in the end. Also, ensure that you do not have any of the fruits and drinks mentioned in the first chapter because these smoothies are not acidic.

Green Alkaline smoothie

Ingredients:

- ☐ 5 frozen strawberries
- ☐ 1 cup of almond milk
- ☐ 1 large handful of fresh spinach
- ☐ 1 cup of water or ice
- ☐ 1 cup of watermelon
- ☐ 1 small banana
- ☐ 1 teaspoon of chia seeds

Nutritional facts:

Calories: 81kcal
Fat: 2g
Sugar: 8g
Carbohydrates: 14g

When you mix vegetables with berries, your smoothie will become brown, and that is something that nobody wants. So, blend your veggies with the banana, chia seeds, and half a cup of water or ice and then blend the remaining ingredients with the strawberries. Berries are acidic by nature, but we need the antioxidants that the berries supply, and that is why we are using non-dairy milk (almond milk) to neutralize the acidity in the berries so that you can get the nutrients without the acidity.

Minty Alkaline Smoothie

Ingredients:

- ☐ ½ kiwi fruit
- ☐ ½ a cup of mint
- ☐ Cucumber
- ☐ 1 banana
- ☐ 2-3 tablespoon of honey
- ☐ Water or almond milk
- ☐ 2 handfuls of Kale
- ☐ ½ cup of lemon juice (optional)

Nutritional facts:

Calories: 180kcal
Fat: 4g
Sugar: 15g
Carbohydrates: 10g

Blend the vegetables first before adding the other ingredients. Lemon is acidic; however, the addition of other alkaline ingredients neutralizes the acidity significantly. Also, lemon juice makes the blood alkaline after it has been metabolized.

Cherry Alkaline Smoothie

Ingredients:

- ☐ 1 cup of almond milk
- ☐ 1 cup of ice (if you need it cold)
- ☐ 1 teaspoon of flax seeds
- ☐ 1 cup of seeded fresh cherries
- ☐ 1 tablespoon of raw cashew
- ☐ ½ a cup of chopped beet

Nutritional facts:

Calories: 170kcal
Fat: 3g
Sugar: 10g
Carbohydrates: 17g

Place all your ingredients in a blender and blend until it is smooth with a cream-like consistency. Although cherries are acidic in nature, they are not only neutralized by the almond milk but act as alkalizing agents after the body has metabolized them.

Boosting Alkaline Smoothie

Ingredients:

- ☐ ½ a cup of coconut milk
- ☐ ¼ cup of cucumber chopped or sliced
- ☐ 1 medium banana
- ☐ 1 handful of spinach or Swiss chard
- ☐ ½ a cup of chopped kiwi fruit
- ☐ ½ cup of water or ice cubes

Nutritional facts:

Calories: 130kcal
Fat: 6g
Sugar: 9g
Carbohydrates: 19g

Blend your ingredients until it is smooth. Going on a diet is not easy, especially if you have not done it before as you are cut off from all the foods and snacks that you would normally eat. Keep going, and by the end of it, you would have achieved all the goals that you had set for yourself.

Banana Alkaline Smoothie

Ingredients:

- ☐ 1 ½ medium size banana
- ☐ ½ cup of blueberries
- ☐ 1 large handful of spinach or alkaline greens powder if there is no spinach
- ☐ 1 teaspoon of flax seeds
- ☐ ½ cup of almond milk
- ☐ ½ cup of water or ice

Nutritional facts:

Calories: 155kcal
Fat: 5g
Sugar: 13g
Carbohydrates: 18g

Blend the greens first with the seeds and a little bit of water, and after you are done, blend the banana and other ingredients. Blend for around 1-2 minutes until your smoothie is smooth with a creamy consistency.

Ginger Alkaline Smoothie

Ingredients:

- ☐ 1 cup of water
- ☐ ½ cup of coconut milk
- ☐ 2 cups of spinach
- ☐ 1 ½ teaspoon of fresh ginger
- ☐ 1 medium-sized banana
- ☐ 1 cup of chopped frozen pineapples (or fresh)
- ☐ ½ a cup of freshly squeezed lemon (optional)

Nutritional facts:

Calories: 181kcal
Fat: 2g
Sugar: 7g
Carbohydrates: 11g

If you do not mind the taste of ginger, you can add one tablespoon of it to your smoothie. Blend the vegetables and water until it is smooth, then blend your banana along with the other ingredients. It is best to drink this smoothie immediately after it has been blended.

Avocado Alkaline Smoothie

Ingredients:

- ☐ 1 large handful of Kale
- ☐ 1 cup of avocado
- ☐ ½ a cup of cucumber
- ☐ 1 teaspoon of chia seeds
- ☐ 1 cup of water
- ☐ 1 cup of almond milk
- ☐ ½ a clove of garlic (optional)
- ☐ 1 small handful of spinach (optional)

Nutritional facts:

Calories: 162kcal
Fat: 12g
Sugar: 3g

Carbohydrates: 16g

If you do not like the taste and smell of garlic, leave it out of your smoothie. Blend the vegetables first, then add the fruits along with the milk and garlic afterward, Blend for 1-2 minutes or until it is smooth.

Kale Alkaline Smoothie

Ingredients:

- ☐ 1 large handful of Kale
- ☐ 1 cup of avocado
- ☐ ½-1 cup of chunks of frozen pineapple
- ☐ 1 tablespoon of ginger (optional)
- ☐ 1 teaspoon of chia seeds
- ☐ 1 medium-size banana
- ☐ ½ cup of cashew
- ☐ 1 cup of almond milk or water

Nutritional facts:

Calories: 172kcal
Fat: 9g
Sugar: 8g
Carbohydrates: 24g

Blend the ingredients starting with the vegetables and a little bit of the almond milk or water until it is smooth. Then, add the remaining ingredients and blend for 1-2 minutes until it is smooth with a creamy consistency

Cucumber Alkaline Smoothie

Ingredients:

- ☐ 1 medium banana
- ☐ 1 cup of almond milk
- ☐ ½ cup of cucumber

- ☐ ½ a cup of water
- ☐ 1 handful of parsley or Kale
- ☐ 1 teaspoon of flax seeds
- ☐ ½ a cup of freshly squeezed lemon juice (optional)

Nutritional facts:

Calories: 171kcal
Fat: 6g
Sugar: 3g
Carbohydrates: 17g

Blend your ingredients starting with the vegetables until it has a smooth or cream-like consistency. You can choose not to add the lemon juice if you do not want to.

Alkaline Pineapple Smoothie

Ingredients:

- ☐ 1 teaspoon of turmeric
- ☐ 1 ½ cup of frozen chunks of pineapple
- ☐ 1 cup of cucumbers
- ☐ ½ a cup of freshly squeezed lemon juice
- ☐ I cup of almond or coconut milk
- ☐ 1 teaspoon of chia seeds
- ☐ 1 cup of ice (if you want your smoothie served cold)

Nutritional facts:

Calories: 151kcal
Fat: 11g
Sugar: 10g
Carbohydrates: 14g

Wash all your ingredients and cut them up before throwing it into the blender. Blend for 1-2 minutes until it is smooth and blend with the ice if you want your smoothie cold. It is best to drink it immediately after blending.

Mango Alkaline Smoothie

Ingredients:

- ☐ 1 cup of spinach
- ☐ 1 handful of kale (optional)
- ☐ ½ tablespoon of fresh ginger
- ☐ 1 cup of mango chunks
- ☐ ½ cup of frozen pineapples
- ☐ 1 teaspoon of chia seeds
- ☐ 1 cup of almond milk
- ☐ 1 cup of ice
- ☐ 1 medium carrot

Nutritional facts:

Calories: 232kcal
Fat: 13g
Sugar: 18g
Carbohydrates: 22g

Add water to it, depending on the consistency that you want. Start blending the vegetables with a little bit of the almond milk until it is smooth, add the remaining ingredients to it and blend for 1-2 minutes.

Vegetable Alkaline Smoothie

Ingredients:

- ☐ 2 medium carrots
- ☐ 1 cucumber
- ☐ 2 handfuls of spinach or Kale
- ☐ ½ a cup of apple
- ☐ 1 cup of water
- ☐ 1 cup of coconut milk
- ☐ I teaspoon of flaxseeds
- ☐ 1 cup of ice (optional)

Nutritional facts:

Calories: 90kcal
Fat: 12g
Sugar: 11g
Carbohydrates: 22g

Wash your ingredients and peel your carrots before putting them in your blender. Remove the core from the apples to avoid seeds getting in and blend the vegetables first before putting in the other ingredients. Blend for 1-2 minutes or until it is smooth with a creamy consistency.

Banana Ginger Alkaline Smoothie

Ingredients:

- ☐ Fresh ginger
- ☐ One banana
- ☐ ¾ vanilla yogurt
- ☐ One tablespoon of honey

Nutritional Facts:

Calories: 157kcal
Fat: 3g
Sugar: 28g
Fiber: 1.5g
Protein: 5g
Carbohydrates: 15g

Wash your ingredients, then throw them into a blender. Afterwards, you blend until you have a deliciously creamy beverage with a cream consistency.

Green Ginger Alkaline Smoothie

Ingredients:

- ☐ 2 teaspoons of hemp seed
- ☐ ¼ cup of fresh lemon juice
- ☐ 3 teaspoons of minced fresh ginger
- ☐ 1 teaspoon of raw honey
- ☐ 2 cups of packed baby spinach
- ☐ 1 ½ cups of ice cubes until smooth

Nutritional Facts:

Calories: 153kcal
Fiber: 4g
Fat: 4g
Sugar: 3g
Sodium: 141mg
Carbohydrates: 11g

Pour all ingredients into a blender and blend until smooth. Divide between 2 glasses and serve.

Apple Crisp Alkaline Smoothie

Ingredients:

- ☐ 2 teaspoon of pecans
- ☐ ¼ teaspoon of cinnamon
- ☐ ¼ cup of old-fashioned rolled oats
- ☐ 1 cup of apple cider
- ☐ ½ cups of 2% vanilla Greek yogurt
- ☐ ¼ teaspoon of nutmeg
- ☐ 1 cup of ice cubes

Nutritional Fact:

Calories: 364kcal
Protein: 14g
Fat: 12.5g
Sugar: 32g
Sodium: 69mg
Carbohydrates: 16g

Gather ingredients in a blender and process until you achieve a creamy consistency, and enjoy.

Berry Breakfast Alkaline Smoothie

Ingredients:

- ☐ One cup of frozen, unsweetened raspberries
- ☐ ¾ cup of chilled unsweetened almond milk
- ☐ ¼ cup of frozen cherries
- ☐ 1 ½ tablespoon honey
- ☐ 2 teaspoons of fresh ginger
- ☐ 1 teaspoon of flaxseed
- ☐ 2 teaspoons of fresh lemon juice

Nutritional Fact:

Calories: 112kcal
Fat: 1.5g
Sodium: 56mg
Sugar: 20g
Fiber: 3g
Protein: 1g
Carbohydrates: 18g

Pure ingredients into a blender and blend until smooth. Afterwards, pour the mixture into two chilled glasses – and there you have your chilled rich breakfast smoothie.

Strawberry-kiwi Alkaline Smoothie

Ingredients:

- ☐ 1 ¼ cup of cold apple juice
- ☐ 1 ripe banana
- ☐ 1 kiwi
- ☐ 5 frozen strawberries
- ☐ 1 ½ teaspoon honey

Nutritional Fact:

Calories: 87kcal
Fat: 0.3g
Sodium: 3.5mg
Sugar: 16.5g
Protein: 0.5g
Fiber: 1.5g
Carbohydrates: 9g

Mix ingredients and blend until desired result is achieved.

Papaya Alkaline Smoothie

Ingredients:

- ☐ 1 papaya
- ☐ Plain yogurt
- ☐ ½ cup fresh pineapple chunks
- ☐ ½ cup crushed ice
- ☐ 1 teaspoon coconut extract
- ☐ 1 teaspoon ground flaxseed

Nutritional Fact:

Calories: 299kcal
Fat: 1.5g
Sugar: 44g
Protein: 13g
Fiber: 7g
Carbohydrates: 19g

Process the ingredient in a blender for about 30 seconds and serve chilled.

Peachy Alkaline Smoothie

Ingredients:

- [ ] One cup of milk
- [ ] 2 teaspoons of vanilla yogurt
- [ ] ½ cup of frozen peaches
- [ ] ½ cup of strawberries
- [ ] 1/8 teaspoon of powdered ginger
- [ ] 2 teaspoons of whey protein powder
- [ ] 3 ice cubes

Nutritional Fact:

Calories: 150kcal
Fat: 2g
Sodium: 73mg
Sugar: 24g
Fiber: 2g
Protein: 9g
Carbohydrates: 14g

If you are not using a high-speed blender, a pro trick is to blend the soft/liquid ingredients together first with the protein powder to ensure even distribution of the protein powder. Having done that, add the harder/solid ingredients, like the fruits and ice, to the blender. Then, you can toss in more ice cubes and serve chilled.

Apricot-Mango Alkaline Smoothie

Ingredients:

- [ ] ¼ teaspoon vanilla extract
- [ ] 8 ice cubes
- [ ] Lemon peel twists
- [ ] 4 teaspoons fresh lemon
- [ ] Low-fat yogurt
- [ ] One cup of milk
- [ ] Six apricot-peeled and chopped-two ripe mango

Nutritional Facts:

Calories: 252kcal

Fat: 3.5 fat
Sugar: 45.5g
Fiber: 6g
Protein: 7g
Sodium: 57mg
Carbohydrates: 15g

Pour ingredients into a blender and blend until cream consistency is achieved.

Watermelon Alkaline Smoothie

Ingredients:

- ☐ 2 cups of chopped watermelon
- ☐ ¼ cup of fat-free milk
- ☐ Tw cups of ice

Nutritional Facts:

Calories: 56kcal
Fat: 0.3g
Sodium: 19.5mg
Fiber: 0.5g
Protein: 2g
Carbohydrates: 7g

Ensure to buy a seedless watermelon or remove seeds from the watermelon before you blend. Blend ingredients for 20 seconds or until you have achieved your desired consistency.

Cranberry Citrus Alkaline Smoothie

Ingredients:

- ☐ 3 oranges peeled
- ☐ ½ cup cranberries
- ☐ ½ banana frozen
- ☐ ¼ cup plain Greek yogurt

☐ ½ teaspoons of vanilla extract

Nutritional Facts:

Calories: 102kcal
Fat: 3g
Sugar: 11g
Sodium: 31mg
Carbohydrate: 11g

Pour ingredients into a blender and blend until you achieve the desired result.

Peanut Butter Banana Alkaline Smoothie

Ingredients:

☐ 2 frozen banana
☐ 2 tablespoons of natural peanut butter
☐ 1 cup of unsweetened milk (nut, soy, animal)
☐ ½ cup of plain Greek yogurt
☐ Honey or maple syrup, to taste

Nutritional Fact:

Calories: 168kcal
Fat: 4g
Carbohydrates: 23g
Sugar: 12g
Sodium: 35mg
Carbohydrates: 18g

Pour all ingredients into a blender and blend until desired consistency is achieved.

Blueberry Alkaline Smoothie

Ingredients:

- [ ] 2 teaspoons of honey
- [ ] 2 cups of milk or almond milk
- [ ] 1 teaspoon of vanilla extract
- [ ] 1 cup of vanilla yogurt or Greek yogurt
- [ ] 2 ½ cups of blueberries, fresh or frozen
- [ ] 1 ½ cup of old-fashioned oats
- [ ] ½ teaspoon of cinnamon
- [ ] Large handful of ice

Nutritional Fact:

Calories: 281kcal
Sugar: 6g
Fat: 5.5g
Protein: 8g
Sodium: 55mg
Carbohydrates: 13g

Pour all ingredients into a blender and blend until desired consistency is achieved.

Banana Mango Avocado Green Alkaline Smoothie

Ingredients:

- [ ] 1 frozen banana
- [ ] 1 cup of frozen mango chunks
- [ ] 1 cup of spinach
- [ ] ½ of medium avocado
- [ ] 1 cup of almond milk or other non-dairy milk
- [ ] 1 cup of vanilla extract
- [ ] Few drops of stevia extract or other sweetener (optional)

Nutritional Fact:

Calories: 198kcal
Fat: 5g
Protein: 6g

Sodium: 40mg
Carbohydrates: 15g

Place all ingredients in a blender and blend until smoothie.

The Banana Green Alkaline Smoothie

Ingredients:

- [ ] 1 cup of kale
- [ ] 1 teaspoon spirulina powder
- [ ] 1 tablespoon of chia seeds
- [ ] ¾ cup of orange juice preferably freshly squeezed
- [ ] ½ cup of fresh mango chunks
- [ ] 1 tablespoon of hemp seeds
- [ ] 1 small-medium banana, peeled or sliced
- [ ] ½ cup of fresh or frozen pineapple chunks

Nutritional Fact:

Calories: 466kcal
Fat: 6g
Sodium: 45mg
Protein: 10g
Carbohydrates: 30g

Place the ingredients, except for the hemp seeds, in a high powered blender and blend until smooth and creamy. Pour blended ingredients into a glass and sprinkle with hemp seeds.

This brings us to the end of this chapter, and I am sure that by the end of the diet, your body would have undergone a complete reset. The smoothies mentioned are completely vegan, sugar-free, and do not contain any dairy products whatsoever. During the course of the diet, make sure to stay away from sugar and processed foods so that your progress would not be hindered.

CHAPTER 4

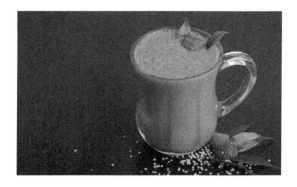

ELECTRIC FOODS

What is the Electric Food Diet?

When we eat, the food that we eat is either healthy or harmful to our body system. Sadly, most of the food we consume do not have nutrients in the proper form for our body to absorb. Generally, most organic foods list nutrients on their nutrients label, but most times, these listed nutrients are not in the proper form for which our body can assimilate. Furthermore, most of our vegetables and fruits are hybrids. These vegetables and fruits simply were made by man. Hybrid foods are high in acidity, which is the opposite of alkalinity. Due to their high level of acidity, hybrid foods cause a disruption in the absorption of nutrients on a cellular level. Therefore, in an attempt to solve this issue of unhealthy and high acidic food consumption by Americans, the idea of electric food was introduced.

Electric foods are foods that are entirely natural, living food indigenous to earth. These foods come from the deep interior of nature, and they remain in their natural state – unchanged by man. The human body is living, and so we need to eat living foods to survive. Electric foods are non-acidic, non-mucus forming, and living foods. Also, electric foods contain alkaline and have an alkaline effect on the body. Unlike other kinds of foods, electric foods can be easily assimilated, broken down, properly digested, utilized, and disposed of by the body. Electric foods are rich in minerals and other rich nutrients that help your body heal from diseases and prevent the outbreak of future diseases. Since the body is created to be naturally electric, it also makes sense to eat electric foods. Now that we understand what electric foods are, the next thing is to explain what an electric food diet is. However, before we proceed, I would like you to take a few minutes to evaluate your health, what you eat, what you drink, and the kind of fruits or vegetables you consume. Having done this evaluation, you may realize that you may have been causing your body more harm than good through what you are eating. The famous Dr. Sebi explained electric food diet had been the root foundation of living a disease-free, non-obese, and addiction-free life. He stressed that the diet was all about minimizing acidity in your food and mucus in your body. Being on an electric food diet means you only eat electric foods that help you develop an alkaline system. This alkaline system built through the electric diet allows your body to fight diseases and prevent the outbreak of future ones. The electric food diet is a culture, a way of life, and a lifestyle. It is not a temporary diet, not something you do only when you are sick or when you want to lose a few pounds. People who are on an electric food diet live a disease-free life. The electric food diet has helped many Americans avoid many of the health hardships prevalent in America today. One importance of the electric food diet is that it helps revitalize your cells by eliminating toxic waste by alkalizing your blood. Electric food entails eating raw foods, sticking to organic and natural foods, and taking a couple of herbal teas and herbal supplements. The electric food diet lacks lactic (diary), uric (meat), or carbonic substances (sugar, salt, and starch).

The human body is naturally made to heal itself, but we can enhance this healing process by feeding it what it needs to operate efficiently and effectively. You don't agree? Or you have doubts. Think about many scratches and scrapes we get that heal on their own without the aid of any medication, orthodox or modern. The electric food diet can be used to restore your body to its natural state and detoxify your body, thereby preventing the outbreak of the disease in your body. The primary bedrock of the electric food diet is education and information. You can start learning about the electric food diet here and then watch out for the change in the trajectory of your health and virtually your life. When you strictly adhere to the electric food diet, you have decided to be healthy and not diseased, be skinny, and not be fat. This one decision is what you need to go from being addicted to being liberated. The electric food diet inculcates in you an alkaline-based lifestyle.

Key Rules of Dr. Sebi's Electric Food Diet

Dr. Sebi's electric food diet has eight main rules that must be adhered to if you want to be healed. These rules practically focus on avoiding animal foods and products, ultra-processed foods, and low protein diet. According to Dr. Sebi's nutritional guide, the following rules are the key rules of the electric food diet:

- ☐ **Rule 1:** You must only eat the food listed in Dr. Sebi's nutritional guide.

- ☐ **Rule 2:** You must drink 1 gallon (3.8 liters) of water every day.

- ☐ **Rule 3:** You must take Dr. Sebi's supplements an hour before medication.

- ☐ **Rule 4:** You are not allowed to take any animal products such as meat or fish.

- ☐ **Rule 5:** You are not allowed to take alcohol.

- ☐ **Rule 6**: The consumption of wheat products is prohibited. You can only consume the natural-growing grains listed in the guide.

- ☐ **Rule 7:** You are not permitted to microwave your food. – Dr. Sebi believes that microwaves kill your food.

- ☐ **Rule 8:** You are not allowed to eat canned or seedless fruits.

Foods Allowed on the Electric Food Diet

Having seen the strict rules of Dr. Sebi's electric food diet, you may be wondering what food you are then allowed to eat. Usually, people think that their food option is limited; well, they are not – Dr. Sebi's electric food diet is basic, simple, and obtainable. Remember that when you feed your body with these foods, you create an internal environment that doesn't harbor disease. Most of the foods, mainly non-hybrid and alkaline-based foods, are highlighted below:

- **Fruits:** Apples, Banana, Orange, Berries (all types, except cranberries), Cantaloupe, Cherries, Figs, Grape (seeded), Limes (key limes, with seed), Mango, Melons (seeded), Papayas, Plums, Peaches, Pears, Prickly pear (cactus fruit), Prunes, Raisins (seeded), Tamarind, Dates, Seville Orange, Soft jelly coconuts, Soursop (Latin or West Indian markets), Tamarind, Elderberries.

- **Vegetables:** Amaranth greens (callaloo, a variety of greens), Avocado, Bell peppers, chayote (Mexican squash), Cucumber, Dandelion greens, Garbanzo beans, Izote (cactus flower/cactus leaf), Kale, Lettuce (all except, iceberg), Mushroom (all except, shitake), Nopales (Mexican cactus), Okra, Olives, Onions, Sea Vegetables (Wakame/dulse/arame/hijiki/nori), Squash, Tomato (cherry and plum only), Tomatillo, Turnip greens, Zucchini, Watercress, Purslane (verdolaga), Wild arugula.

- **Grains:** Amaranth, Fonio, Kamut, Quinoa, Rye, Spelt, Tef, Wild rice.

- **Natural Herbal Teas:** Burdock, Chamomile, Elderberry, Fennel, Ginger, Raspberry, Tila.

- **Oils:** Olive oil (avoid cooking it), Coconut oil (cooking it is prohibited), Grapeseed oil, Sesame oil, Hemp Seed oil, and Avocado oil.

- **Nuts & Seeds (including Nuts & Seed Butters):** Hemp seeds, Raw sesame seeds, Raw sesame "tahini" butter, Brazil nuts.

- **Spices & Seasonings:**

  - ☐ *Mild Flavours:* Basil, Bay leaf, Cloves, Dill, Oregano, Savory, Sweet basil, Tarragon, Thyme.

  - ☐ *Sweet Flavours (Natural Sweeteners):* Pure Agave Syrup (from cactus), Date sugar.

  - ☐ *Pungent & Spicy Flavours:* Achiote, Cayenne/African Bird pepper, Onion Powder, Habanero, and Sage.

  - ☐ Salt Flavours: Pure Sea Salt, Powdered Granulated Seaweed, kelp/dulse/nori – with sea taste.

Note: If a food is not listed above, then it is not recommended. Also, while natural growing grains are alkaline-based; it is highly proffered that you consume only the grains listed above, and not consume wheat. Finally, most of the foods, especially the grains, listed above, are available as pasta, bread, and flour or cereals and can be easily purchased at better health food stores. In any case, foods consisting of yeast or baking powder are prohibited.

Other foods you may be permitted to eat on the electric diet.

Since the electric food diet emphasizes the consumption of nutrient-rich vegetables, fruits, whole grains, and healthy oils, the following are other foods you may be permitted to eat on the electric diet:

- Chia seed
- Quinoa
- Ethiopian teff
- Watermelon (strictly the ones with seeds)

- Sprouts – alfalfa, flax, wheatgrass
- Cabbages
- Coconut

Foods that are not Permitted on this Diet

If any food is not included in Dr. Sebi's Nutritional guide, then such food is not permitted on this diet. Example of such foods are:

- Canned fruits or vegetables
- Hybridized foods
- Eggs
- Dairy (milk)
- Fish
- Red Meat
- Poultry
- Soya Products
- Processed or packaged foods, restaurant take-outs are not excluded.
- Wheat
- Alcohol
- Yeast or foods leavened with yeast
- Baking powder or foods leavened with baking powder.
- Carbonic acids such as salt, sugar (except date sugar and agave syrup), and starch.
- Man-made/hybridized foods
- Seedless fruits
- Carrots
- Broccoli

Finally, many vegetables, fruits, grains, nuts, and seeds are banned on the electric food diet. Therefore, if a vegetable, grain, fruit, nut, or seed isn't listed above, it may not be eaten during the electric food diet.

Electric Herbs

If you have resolutely resolved to embark on this journey to healthier living, then electric herbs and smoothie are for you. Electric herbs serve as both food and nourishment for the human body and play a huge role in detoxing the human system. The lack of proper exercise and proper nutrition in the body results in harm for the body. Therefore, electric herbs serve as a panacea by providing the body with the needed and essential nutrients through vegetables, fruits, and plant minerals. All of them were living products and fed to the human body, which is also a living thing. Some of these electric herbs include:

1. **Red Willow Bark:** Most, if not all, of the commercial aspirins out there today was extracted from this medicinal herb. This electric herb contains iron-phosphate, calcium, magnesium, and potassium. If you have ever heard Dr. Sebi speak of Cancasha, this is the Cancasha he spoke of. This electric herb is used to cure headaches in adults. Note, however – they cannot be used by pregnant women.

2. **Irish moss:** Is an excellent all-rounder rich in minerals and vegetables. It is also referred to as Sea moss by Dr. Sebi. They can be consumed by people of all ages, and also by pregnant women. They are best consumed raw and wild-crafted.

3. **Burdock Root:** This herb, when prepared as tea, provides all 102 minerals the body is made of. Also, this iron-rich tea can be consumed by people of all ages and pregnant women. Additionally, this herb, when prepared as cooled tea, can be used externally to cure all kinds of skin conditions.

4. **Yellow dock Root:** If you are looking for an electric herb for blood cleansing, then Yellow dock root is your best bet. They can be used by people of all ages; however, they are a no-go for pregnant ladies.

5. **Elderberry:** This electric herb is an excellent choice for an anti-inflammatory and antioxidant electric herb. This herb is an excellent source of phosphorus, iron, potassium, and copper. They can be used by people of all ages, and also by pregnant women.

6. **Other electric herbs:** Basil, Moringa, Cayenne Pepper, Sage, Red Clover, Plantain, Dandelion, Oregano, Thyme, and Sarsaparilla.

CHAPTER 5

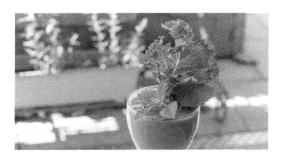

HEALTH BENEFITS OF THE ELECTRIC SMOOTHIE DIET

Like I mentioned in the previous chapter, electric food is natural, indigenous, "live" foods that promote positive changes for a healthy living. Electric foods are leavened with enzymes and beneficial nutrients. The fresher the electric foods you consume are, the more likely it is for you to get these life-transforming and life-giving nutrients. At this juncture, I am assuming that you have commenced your electric food lifestyle, and you are beginning to think, "What exactly are the benefits of the electric smoothie diet?" The answers to the question will be exhaustively provided in this chapter. Keep reading.

One of the benefits of the electric smoothie diet is its immense promotion of plant-based foods. This diet emphasizes the consumption of vegetables and fruits, which have been associated with reduced inflammation and oxidant stress, as well as protection against many diseases. These vegetables and fruits are high in fiber, minerals, plant compounds, and vitamins.

- **Restore your alkaline state:**
  The electric smoothie diet helps improve your body's alkaline state. This diet helps your body maintain its blood pH level. A pH level is how you measure how

acidic or alkaline a thing is. When the pH level of a substance is at 0-6 level, then that thing is acidic. However, when the pH level is 8-14, then that substance is completely alkaline. Note that when the pH level is at 7, the pH level is neutral. Therefore, what an electric smoothie diet does is promote plant-based and alkaline-based foods. This diet emphasizes fruits and vegetables that are rich in alkaline. So when this diet is strictly adhered to by a person, he/she promotes the alkalinity level in their body system and reduces the acidity level. While alkalinity is good for the body, acidity is toxic to the human body system. This diet also helps your body maintain its blood pH level.

- **Detoxify your body:**
  When your body is being detoxified, harmful toxins in your body are extracted. Using the electric smoothie diet to detoxify your body, does a lot of wonder to your body. Since electric foods are high in alkaline and discourage the consumption of hybrid or fortified foods, it is a great choice for the detoxification of the body. When detoxifying the body, you swap caffeinated drinks like tea or coffee for green tea. You, of course, know by now that green tea is an electric food. Fruits and vegetables that are used for the electric smoothie diet are loaded with essential fibers that aid digestion. Cinnamon and fenugreek tea that boost body metabolism are used to detoxify the human body.

- **Cure anemia:**
  Sickle cell anemia is caused by the lack of iron fluorine. You can get sufficient iron phosphate from the electric smoothie diet. The highest concentration of iron fluorine is found in the sarsaparilla root. Other electric herbs with high iron fluorine concentration include: burdock root, cocolmeca, elderberry, nettle, and yellow dock root.

- **Treat leukemia and lupus:**
  By choosing to eat healthier food, eating more fresh fruits and vegetables, eating "live and unprocessed foods, exercising and meditating, these diseases can be healed and reverted.

- **Revert diabetes:**
  Electric smoothie diets discourage the consumption of sugar and starch; hence it can be used to revert diabetes, which is caused by sugar. Consumption of sugar promotes acidity in the body. This acidity, in turn, fosters toxicity and the prevalence of diabetes and other diseases in the body.

- **Clears Pneumonia:**
  Is a respiratory infection that affects your lungs, thereby preventing sufficient oxygen from getting to your bloodstream. The electric smoothie diet discourages the use of dairy products that cause mucus.

Other Health Benefits

Asides the health benefits of the electric smoothie diet highlighted earlier, some other health benefits of the electric smoothie diet are:

- Reduced inflammation stress
- Reduced oxidant stress
- Lowers the incidence of heart disease
- Reduces the rate of cancer diet
- Reduces the risk of heart disease
- Improved diet quality
- Healthy weight loss
- Prevents kidney stones
- Keep bones and muscles fit and strong
- Improved brain function

In conclusion, the electric smoothie diet increases the alkaline in the body and reduces the body's acidity. When the smoothie diet is taken early in the morning, it goes directly into the bloodstream, and the nutrients in the smoothie diet naturally cleanse the liver, kidneys, blood, lungs, and digestive tract.

Mistakes to Avoid During Smoothie Preparation

Smoothies are a healthy addition you can make to your diet but if not done properly you won't reap the benefits that you seek. Making a smoothie is more than just blending a bunch of fruits and vegetables together because with a few mistakes, you can end up with a bunch of sugars and none of the nutrients you wanted. For the perfect smoothie, avoid these mistakes:

- **Adding too much fruits:** Fruits have a lot of nutrients but they do have calories as well and if you put them together, you might end up consuming more calories than you expected. Plus, fruits tend to have a lot of sugar so you need to be cautious of the fruits you put in your smoothies.

- **Forgetting to add protein:** The main essence of going on a smoothie diet or including it in your lifestyle is to have access to a lot of nutrients without necessarily eating a full meal, so this purpose is defeated if there is no protein in your smoothie. You can add items such as chia seeds, soy milk, nut butters, nuts, Greek yoghurt, and oats to your smoothie since they are rich in protein. Plus, the proteins help to keep you feeling full for longer hours which helps to curb your appetite.

- **Forgetting portions:** Like food, you can't forget that portion size plays a huge role on the amount of calories that you consume. If you put a bunch of items together and fill your blender up, you might end up consuming more calories than you normally would in a single sitting. Take your time to measure the fruits, vegetables and other items before blending it into a smoothie.

- **Keeping your fruits and vegetables for too long:** When buying the items you need for a smoothie, buy it in small portions that would last at least a week rather than buying something that could last till the end of your diet. When you store your fruits and vegetables in the fridge for too long, the nutrients slowly begin to decrease and might get destroyed all together so when you blend it, all you get is sugars. Also, do not blend everything you have and store it as smoothies for a long time but do enough that you can drink immediately.

- **Forgetting to make it balanced:** Smoothies are not all about fruits as there are other ingredients that make it one of the healthiest drinks you can take. Include vegetables, whole grains, nuts, seeds, dairy products etc. so that you can get the nutrients and reap the benefits all in one drink.

- **Forgetting to add fiber:** when buying ingredients you need for your smoothie, ensure you purchase fiber. Fiber is what helps you to feel full and prevents you from feeling hungry. Without any fiber in your smoothie, you risk consuming or craving a lot of unwanted junks throughout the day. Therefore, you include fruits that are rich in fiber in your smoothie ingredient.

- **Adding more sweetener:** including a teaspoon of maple syrup or honey in your smoothie add at least 60 calories to your smoothie. With the right recipe you should get enough sweetness with the fruits or flavorings used. For sweetness, you should consider adding raisins, dates or prunes to your smoothie. You can also add spices for additional taste like cinnamon, all spice, or nutmeg. However, when you are just starting out on a smoothie detox, it will take a while for your body to adjust to the lack of sugar but stick to the diet anyways.

- **Forgetting to add the greens:** green are not only easy to prepare but they also taste great. Smoothies that contain greens are packed with vital nutrients and the easiest way to increase your daily vegetable intake. Whether you add green powder or fresh greens like kale, spinach or watercress to your smoothies, you are consuming vegetable intake. However, fresh greens are far more nutritious than green powder. More so, recent studies have shown that watercress is the most nutrient dense food. When preparing your next smoothie, make sure that at least 1/3 of the ingredients (by size) are green vegetables. I recommend spinach because it does a lot of great work in smoothies and it has a mild taste with a lot of vitamins.

- **Using too much ice:** using too many ice cubes makes it harder for the good fats from flax oil, coconut oil, seed or nuts to get incorporated into your glass of smoothie. Henceforth, make sure you add ice last, to ensure that every ingredient and its nutrients are well-incorporated and that you have control over the ratio of cubes to beverage. One good alternative however is that you freeze leftover coconut milk or almond milk in an ice tray, and use those cubes instead of frozen water cubes for your next smoothie.

- **Using under-ripe fruits:** if you wouldn't eat plain under-ripe fruits on a normal day, then why would you prepare your smoothie with under-ripe fruits? First, an under-ripe fruit is hard so it wouldn't blend well. Second, an under-ripe fruit wouldn't taste good. On the flip side, ripe fruits, whether bruised or unbruised is always a great choice because of the taste.

- **Adding all the liquid once:** pouring/dumping all of your milk, juice, coconut milk/water or almond milk right away could result in you having a too-thin smoothie. So what you should do is this: blend in half the liquid first, then add your greens, fruits, seeds, nuts, oil, then ice and see if you like the consistency.

Some make these mistakes without knowing it and since they are not aware of the mistakes they are making, they wouldn't be able to find a solution if it hinders their progress. Make sure you measure every ingredient you use in your smoothie so that you won't eat a lot of sugars with no nutrients without realizing it.

CHAPTER 6

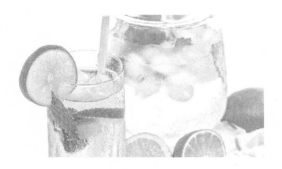

DELICIOUS ELECTRIC FOOD SMOOTHIES

At this juncture, you must have gathered sufficient information on the health benefits of electric food smoothies; it is time to learn how to make those delicious electric food smoothie recipes. This chapter will discuss some smoothies that are ideal for your electric food diet. These smoothies contain amazing nutrients that can help cleanse body organs such as the liver, kidneys, and blood. These smoothies are made with natural, non-hybrid fruits and vegetables – and this is the kind of smoothie your body needs.

Electric Berry Sea Moss Smoothie

Ingredients:

- ☐ ½ cup of greens
- ☐ One lime (freshly squeezed)
- ☐ 1 cup of ice (if you want it cold/chilled)
- ☐ ½ cup mixed berries
- ☐ ½ banana (frozen)
- ☐ Coconut water, 1 cup
- ☐ 1 tablespoon of sea moss

Nutritional facts:

Calories: 80kcal
Carbs: 4g
Fat:2g
Carbohydrates: 12g

Directions/Instruction: starting with the green, blend for one to two minutes. It is better to blend the greens alone first to avoid a brown smoothie. Afterward, add all other ingredients and blend all together until smooth.

Electric Raspberry Greens Smoothie

Ingredients:

- [ ] 1 cup of frozen raspberry
- [ ] 2 teaspoons of lime juice
- [ ] 1 cup of coconut milk
- [ ] 1 handful leafy greens
- [ ] 1 cup of ice (if you want it cold)
- [ ] 1 teaspoon of sea moss

Nutritional facts:

Calories: 150kcal
Carbs: 10g
Fat:4g
Carbohydrates: 17g

Directions/Instructions: make sure you blend the vegetables first before you add other ingredients. Lime is the chief alkaline ingredient in this smoothie. Hence it must be included in the smoothie. Keep blending until all the ingredients have blended smoothly.

Electric Mango-Banana Smoothie

Ingredients:

- ☐ ½ banana
- ☐ 1 cup of water
- ☐ 2 cups of greens
- ☐ 1 mango
- ☐ 1 cup of ice (if you want it cold)

Nutritional facts:

Calories: 155kcal
Carbs: 13g
Fat: 5g
Carbohydrates: 20g

Directions/Instructions: blend your smoothie ingredients. Even though the electric food smoothie diet voyage might not be all rosy – you can't eat any of your favorite foods and snacks anymore. However, do not back down, keep your heads up and keep going until you have smashed the goals you set for yourself.

Electric Sea Moss Green Smoothie

Ingredients:

- ☐ 2 full teaspoons of sea moss
- ☐ 2 cups mixed greens
- ☐ One banana
- ☐ 1 cup of ice (if you want it cold)

Nutritional facts:

Calories: 162kcal
Carbs: 12g
Fat: 2g
Carbohydrates: 11g

Directions/Instructions: blend all ingredients until smooth. You can decide to add a few cubes or a cup of ice to your smoothie, and you might not add ice cubes at all – it is your choice to make. However, it is essential to state that some smoothies are better served chilled.

Electric Kale Berry Smoothie

Ingredients:

- ☐ 1 cup of water or 1 cup of coconut or 1 cup of nut milk
- ☐ One large apple
- ☐ 2 cups of kale
- ☐ 1 cup of mixed berries

Nutritional facts:

Calories: 172kcal
Carbs:24g
Fat:3g
Carbohydrates: 26g

Directions/Instructions: make sure to blend all ingredients until they have been smoothly blended. For this smoothie, you can use either a cup of water, a coconut, or a cup of nut milk.

Electric Apple Juice Smoothie

Ingredients:

- ☐ 1 peeled apple
- ☐ 2 cups of steamed kale
- ☐ ½ avocado
- ☐ 1 ½ cups of apple juice

Nutritional facts:

Calories: 150kcal
Carbs: 10g
Fat:11g
Carbohydrates: 16g

Directions/Instructions: carefully arrange all your ingredients in your blender and blend until all the ingredients have been smoothly blended.

Electric Banana Flax Smoothie

Ingredients:

- ☐ ½ cup of blueberries
- ☐ 1 banana (frozen)
- ☐ 1 cup of water
- ☐ 1 teaspoon of flax seeds
- ☐ 2 cups greens

Nutritional facts:

Calories: 230kcal
Carbs: 22g
Fat:15g
Carbohydrates: 24g

Direction/Instruction: place your ingredients in a high powered blender and blend until your smoothie has a creamy consistency.

Electric Green Smoothie

Ingredients:

- ☐ 1 cup of coconut water or a cup of filtered water
- ☐ ½ lime (peeled)
- ☐ 1-inch fresh ginger
- ☐ 1 date
- ☐ 1 handful of greens
- ☐ ½ cucumber (peeled)
- ☐ 1 cup of water

Nutritional facts:

Calories: 200kcal
Carbs: 23g
Fat: 14g
Carbohydrates: 20g

Directions/Instructions: first, you blend your greens with water or milk before you add other ingredients. This is done to avoid a brown smoothie – no one wants a brown smoothie. Now, meticulously arrange the rest of your ingredients in a high powered blender and blend until your smoothie has smoothly blended.

Electric Apple Berries Smoothie

Ingredients:

- ☐ 1 cup water or 1 cup of hemp milk (a cup of ice can also be added if you want it cold)
- ☐ 1 large apple
- ☐ 2 cups greens
- ☐ 1 cup of mixed berries (this mixture may include: raspberries, strawberries, and blueberries)

Nutritional facts:

Calories: 90kcal
Carbs: 14g
Fat: 11g
Carbohydrates: 22g

Directions/Instructions: you must first blend your greens separately to avoid creating a brown smoothie. Afterward, carefully arrange the rest of the ingredients in your blender (preferably a high powered blender) and blend until all of the ingredients are perfectly blended.

Electric Banana Berry Kale Smoothie

Ingredients:

- ☐ 1 banana
- ☐ 1 cup of strawberries (could be fresh or frozen)
- ☐ 1 cup of ice
- ☐ 1 cup of chopped kale

Nutritional facts:

Calories: 171kcal
Carbs: 12g
Fat: 6g
Carbohydrates: 16g

Directions/Instructions: meticulously place the ingredients in your high powered blender and blend until a desired creamy consistency is achieved.

Electric Banana Coconut Smoothie

Ingredients:

- ☐ 1 pear
- ☐ 1 banana
- ☐ 1 cup of coconut water
- ☐ 2 cups of kale (preferably chopped kale)
- ☐ 1 cup of ice (if you desire to serve smoothie chilled)

Nutritional facts:

Calories: 200kcal
Carbs: 22g
Fat: 12g
Carbohydrates: 24g

Directions/Instructions: to get the best out of this smoothie, make sure to carefully place the ingredients mentioned above in a high-powered blender and blend it to satisfaction. Remember that the kale must be chopped to get the best nutritional effect of this smoothie.

Electric Banana Berries Smoothie

Ingredients:

- ☐ 1 handful of watercress
- ☐ ½ cup of blueberries
- ☐ Three baby bananas
- ☐ 1 thumb ginger
- ☐ 2 cups of springs or coconut water
- ☐ ¼ cup of lime juice
- ☐ 1 tablespoon of burdock root powder
- ☐ 6 dates
- ☐ 1 cup of ice (if you want to serve chilled or cold)

Nutritional facts:

Calories: 172kcal
Carbs: 20g
Fat: 9g
Carbohydrates: 28g

Directions/Instructions: carefully arrange and combine all the ingredients into a blender. Then, proceed to blend for two minutes or more. The most important thing is for all the ingredients to be completely mixed into a thick drink. You can add a cup of ice if you want to serve cold or chilled.

Electric Milk and Honey Smoothie

Ingredients:

- ☐ 1 ½ cups of unsweetened almond milk
- ☐ 1 medium-sized Kirby cucumber (peeled and sliced)
- ☐ 1 cup seedless green grapes
- ☐ 2 medium stalks celery (peeled and sliced)
- ☐ 1 teaspoon of honey

Nutritional Facts:

Calories: 124kcal
Fat: 2g
Protein: 2g
Sodium: 170mg
Carbohydrates: 26g
Sugar: 21g (9g added sugar)
Fiber: 2g

Blend until the mixture is smooth.

Electric Pineapple Smoothie

Ingredients:

- ☐ 1 cup of low fat or light vanilla yogurt
- ☐ 6 ice cubes
- ☐ 1 cup of pineapple chunks

Nutritional Fact:

Calories: 280kcal
Fat: 3.5g
Sodium: 167mg
Carbs: 53.5g
Fiber: 2g
Protein: 13g
Sugar: 48g

Place all the ingredients into a blender and pulse as needed, or until the mixture is smooth.

Electric Peaches and Oatmeal Smoothie

Ingredients:

- ☐ ½ cup of whole milk
- ☐ ½ cup of Greek yogurt
- ☐ ½ cup of rolled oats
- ☐ ½ of fresh frozen banana

- ☐ ½ cup of ice cube
- ☐ 1 cup of frozen peaches

Nutritional Facts:

Calories: 217kcal
Fat: 5.5g
Protein: 11g
Sodium: 47mg
Carbohydrates: 33g
Sugar: 15g
Fiber: 4g

Blend ingredients in a blender until smooth.

Electric Banana-Blueberry-Soy Smoothie

Ingredients:

- ☐ 1 ¼ cups of light soy milk
- ☐ ½ cup frozen blueberries
- ☐ ½ frozen banana
- ☐ 1 teaspoon of pure vanilla extract

Nutritional Facts:

Calories: 125kcal
Fat: 1.5g
Sodium: 60mg
Carbs: 25g
Sugar: 11g
Fiber: 2g
Protein: 3g

Combine the ingredients and blend for 20 to 30 seconds until desired creamy consistency is achieved.

Electric Citrus-Pineapple Smoothie

Ingredients:

- [ ] ½ cup fat-free Greek yogurt
- [ ] ½ cup of frozen pineapple chunks
- [ ] 1 teaspoon of vanilla extract
- [ ] ½ navel orange
- [ ] ½ ruby grapefruit

Nutritional Fact:

Calories: 240kcal
Fat: 8g
Protein: 12g
Sodium: 34mg
Carbohydrates: 31g
Fiber: 5g

Pour all ingredients into a blender and blend mixture until desired smoothness is achieved.

Electric Pear-Spinach Smoothie

Ingredients:

- [ ] 1 cup of spinach
- [ ] ¾ cup of Greek yogurt
- [ ] 1 Bartlett pear
- [ ] ½ piece ginger
- [ ] A handful of ice

Nutritional facts:

Calories: 140kcal
Fat: 3g
Protein: 6g
Carbohydrate: 30g
Fiber: 3g

Blend spinach first, then blend other ingredients until desired creamy consistency is achieved.

Electric Chia Seed Green Smoothie

Ingredients:

- ☐ 1 cup of spinach
- ☐ 1 cup unsweetened almond milk
- ☐ 1 cup of frozen pineapple chunks
- ☐ 1 banana
- ☐ 1 teaspoon of chia seeds

Nutritional fact:

Calories: 290kcal
Fat: 5g
Fiber: 2g
Carbohydrate: 25
Carbs: 21

Combine all ingredients, then pour into your blend until you achieve desired smoothness.

Electric Carrot Smoothie

Ingredients:

- ☐ 1 cup of chopped carrots
- ☐ ½ cup of frozen sliced banana
- ☐ Pinch nutmeg
- ☐ ½ cup of unsweetened vanilla almond milk
- ☐ 2 teaspoons of toasted walnut
- ☐ ¼ teaspoon of cinnamon
- ☐ ¼ cup of frozen diced pineapple
- ☐ ½ cup of plain Greek yogurt
- ☐ 1 tablespoon of flaked coconut

Nutritional Fact:

Calories: 320

Fat: 2g
Carbs: 39g
Sodium: 89mg
Carbohydrates: 55g

Add all of your ingredients to the blender, then blend until desired smoothness is achieved. Serve with toppings such as shredded carrots, coconuts or walnuts.

Electric Pumpkin Coconut Smoothie

Ingredients:

- ☐ 2 teaspoons of pumpkin pie
- ☐ 1 cup of ice
- ☐ 1 cup of coconut milk
- ☐ ¼ cup organic pumpkin pie spice
- ☐ 1 frozen sliced banana

Nutritional Fact:

Calories: 292kcal
Carbohydrates: 20g
Protein: 3g
Fat: 24g
Sugar: 8g
Fiber: 2g

Blend all ingredients until creamy consistency is achieved.

Electric Blueberry Almond Smoothie

Ingredients:

- ☐ 1 cup of almond milk
- ☐ ½ cup of frozen blueberries
- ☐ ½ cup of whole wheat grains
- ☐ 1 frozen banana

Nutritional Fact:

Calories: 350kcal
Fat: 3.5g
Sugar: 44g
Fiber: 7g
Protein: 9g
Carbs: 74g

Pour all ingredients into the blender, blend continuously for 20 seconds. Then scrape down the side and blend for an additional 15 seconds.

Electric Tangerine-honey Smoothie

Ingredients:

- ☐ 4 tangerines
- ☐ 2 limes
- ☐ ¼ cup of honey
- ☐ 1 cup of ice

Nutritional Fact:

Calories: 122kcal
Fat: 4g
Protein: 6g
Sodium: 31mg
Carbs: 14g

Pour all ingredients into a blender and blend until desired consistency is achieved.

Electric Peach-ginger Smoothie

Ingredients:

- ☐ 2 cups of frozen sliced peaches
- ☐ 1 ½ cups of buttermilk

- ☐ 3 tablespoons of brown sugar
- ☐ 1 tablespoon of grated fresh ginger

Nutritional Fact:

Calories: 301kcal
Fat: 5g
Protein: 7g
Sodium: 40mg
Carbs: 35g

Pour all ingredients into a blender and blend until desired consistency is achieved.

Electric Pineapple-coconut

Ingredients:

- ☐ 2 cups of coconut water in 1 or 2 ice-cube trays
- ☐ 2 cups of chopped pineapples
- ☐ 1 ½ tablespoons of lime juice
- ☐ 1 tablespoon of honey
- ☐ ½ cup of coconut water

Nutritional Facts:

- ☐ Calories: 255kcal
- ☐ Fat: 5g
- ☐ Protein: 2g
- ☐ Sodium: 23mg
- ☐ Carbs: 23g

Pour all ingredients into a blender and blend until desired consistency is achieved.

Electric Apple-Ginger Smoothie

Ingredients:

- ☐ 1 chopped apple
- ☐ ½ inch of peeled ginger
- ☐ 2 cups of lime juice
- ☐ ¼ cup of honey
- ☐ 1 cup of water
- ☐ 2 cups of ice cubes

Nutritional Fact:

Calories: 140kcal
Fat: 6g
Carbs: 34g
Sodium: 51mg
Protein: 8g

Pour all ingredients into a blender and blend until desired consistency is achieved.

Electric Cucumber-kale Smoothie

Ingredients:

- ☐ 1 ¼ cups of vegetable juice
- ☐ ½ peeled cucumber
- ☐ 3 kale leaves
- ☐ ½ cup of lemon juice

Nutritional Fact:

Calories: 132kcal
Protein: 4g
Fat: 2g
Carbs:51g
Sodium: 40mg

Pour all ingredients into a blender and blend until desired consistency is achieved.

BONUS CONTENT

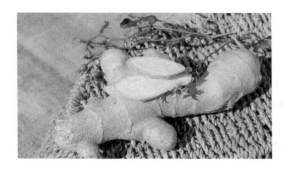

Dr. SEBI'S MEDICINAL HERBAL PLANTS

Dr. Sebi's Medicinal Herbal Plants

- ☐ Basil leaves
- ☐ Turmeric
- ☐ Ginger
- ☐ Mint
- ☐ Cinnamon
- ☐ Chamomile
- ☐ Evening primrose oil
- ☐ Tea tree oil
- ☐ Echinacea
- ☐ Grape seed extract
- ☐ Lavender

Top 19 Medicinal Herbal Plants and its recommended Uses

In this century, we live in a world where manufactured, and processed medicines are prevalent. However, that doesn't mean that herbal medicines cannot be used as an alternative for healing and treatment. After all, herbal medicinal plants are the genesis of how medication started. Also, herbal medicinal plants have the ability to heal, treat, remedy and boost physical and mental fitness or well-being. While it is a known fact that these processed and manufactured medicines have become an integral part of this generation, it can be relieving and soothing to know that we can also approach nature for the power of healing and treatment. These herbal medicinal plants are available as an alternative and complement to our modern health practices and medications. If you would like to add some herbal medicinal plants to your medicinal lifestyle, then I hope this bonus section arms you with sufficient knowledge to start your herbal medicinal plant voyage. Here are ten medicinal herbal plants and its recommended uses:

1. **Turmeric:** Originally from India, turmeric is believed to have anticancer elements and can prevent DNA mutations. This herb can also be used as an anti-inflammatory for older adults who have arthritis. Furthermore, recent studies and research have shown that turmeric is a prospective treatment for various dermatologic diseases and joint diseases such as arthritis. When it comes to culinary functions, turmeric can be used as a cooking ingredient. It is a delicious, antioxidant-rich ingredient to an array of many dishes. This medicinal herbal plant is best consumed when ingested as an herb in cooking or tea. Short-term use is highly recommended – long term use can potentially result in stomach complications. Turmeric has been used as a medicinal herbal plant for over 4, 000 years.

2. **Aloe Vera:** This medicinal herbal plant is popularly known as the 'king of medicinal herbal plant.' Aloe Vera is well-known for its ability to survive in extremely dry conditions as it contains water in its fleshy leaves. Aloe Vera is renowned as a cure to a wide variety of health issues, such as Acne, Constipation, Poor Immune system, Digestive issues.

3. **Flaxseed:** If you are looking for a safe choice for dietary supplements among medicinal herbal plants, then the flaxseed is your go-to. Although subjected to further research and studies, one researcher once asserted that flaxseed could be used to prevent colon

cancer. However, today, flaxseed is recognized as a go-to medicinal herb for its antioxidant effect and anti-inflammatory advantages. Another research claims that flaxseed, when consumed, can aid the reduction of obesity. Flaxseeds are available in oil, flour, and tablets, and can be added to oatmeal and smoothies. For plant-based sources for fatty acids, flax seeds are your best bet. To avoid the toxic effect of the flaxseed, do not consume raw or unripe flaxseed.

4. **Gingko:** Is a key medicinal herbal plant in the Chinese and Asian medical world in general. This herbal plant is the oldest medicinal herbal plant, and the leaves are used by modern medical practitioners to create capsules, tablets, and extracts. While traditionally, ginkgo is consumed as a tea. Studies claim that this herb boost brain health treats patients with moderate dementia, and can influence bone healing. When ingested, ginkgo seeds can be poisonous to the human body.

5. **Tulsi:** In the Hindu religion, this herbal plant has huge religious significance. Besides that, this herbal plant has the ability to keep bacterial growth at bay. Tulsi is known for its strong aroma, and it can be used to: promote longevity, treat cough, treat heart diseases and diabetes, fight stress, and take care of digestion issues.

6. **Mint:** Mint is known for its fragrant, which serves an array of functions. Amongst other things, mint enhances the digestion process and helps lighten your mood. However, for this medicinal plant to thrive, it needs a lot of watering. Another interesting thing about this herb is that, when you plant it in your home garden, its fragrance oozes the ability to chase pets and insects so your home and garden environments will be pest and insect free. Mint is also lauded for its ability to repel cough, boost the immune system, and keep mosquitoes away.

7. **Ginger:** Ginger is widely regarded as a solution to a lot of health problems. In fact, in Indian, ginger, due to its flavor, is an ingredient of Indian foods. Recent research claims that ginger can be used to relieve menstrual pains and cramps. Asides this, ginger can also be used to cure indigestion, cold, flu, asthma, and control blood pressure.

8. **Chamomile:** Chamomile is another great herbal plant that is believed to contain anti-anxiety components. According to a recently published survey, over a million cups of chamomile tea are drunk around the world daily. However, chamomile can also be ingested through capsules, liquids, tablets. If you are looking to treat extreme anxiety disorder cases, then chamomile is a superior solution. Chamomile also has the ability to relieve you from stress and insomnia.

9. **Fennel:** Fennel, also called, saunf, is a medicinal plant with an aromatic flavor. When consumed, fennel is believed to improve eyesight. Fennel seed is a popular herbal plant among Indians – they chew these seeds after eating. Fennel is used to cure cough, control cholesterol, cure, acidity, and improve breast milk supply for women lactating.

10. **Coriander:** Is a medicinal herbal plant that basically can also be used as an ingredient in the kitchen. All its components – seeds, leaves, and powder – have health benefits. These benefits include; improved digestion, treats acne, rich in antioxidants, and cures urine retention.

11. **Tea tree oil:** tea tree oil is a medicinal herbal plant also referred to as melaleuca oil. Tea tree oil has been used as a traditional medicine by aborigines for centuries. This medicinal plant is an essential oil distilled from the leaves of an Australian tea tree called Melaleuca alternifolia. This oil when distilled contains antibacterial, antiviral, antifungal and anti-inflammatory properties. This medicinal plant can be

used to treat acne, athlete's foot, contact dermatitis or head lice. This medicinal plant should never be swallowed. Some people even use the tea tree oil as a natural hand sanitizer as it aids the killing of a number of germs responsible for cold flu, and other illnesses. Tea tree oil can be used as an efficient and safe deodorant as it is known to contain compounds that fight bacteria responsible for body odour. If your skin is sensitive, make sure you mix tea tree oil with an equal amount of coconut oil, olive oil or almond oil.

12. **Echinacea:** Echinacea, also referred to as purple coneflower, is one of the most renowned medicinal herbal plants in the world today. This herbal plant is a group of flowering plants used as a popular herbal remedy. This medicinal herbal plant is believed to possess supplements that boosts the immune system. This medicinal herbal plant is used to support a range of diseases such as, coughs and cold, bronchitis, gingivitis, influenza, canker sores, yeast infection, ear infection, vaginitis, some inflammatory conditions and upper respiratory infections. Echinacea can be found in the following forms: teas, pills, herbal preparation used for skin, juice when squeezed and as an extract in capsules.

13. **Grape seed extract:** this herbal plant is a dietary supplement derived by removing, drying and pulverizing the bitter-tasting seeds of the grape fruit. Grape seed extract is one of the best sources of proanthocyanidins. With the presence of antioxidant compounds, this medicinal herbal plant is used to fight illnesses and safeguard the body against oxidative stress, tissue damage and all forms of inflammation. Grape seed extract has the following health benefits: cardiovascular benefits, protection against pathogens, improved night vision, prevention against skin cancer, improved bone strength, aids healing of wounds and prevents cognitive decline. Note however that grape seed extract should not be administered to pregnant women.

14. **Lavender:** lavender is a medicinal herbal plant originally located in northern Africa and the mountain regions of the Mediterranean. This herbal plant is highly renowned for skin and beauty purposes – it is commonly used in fragrances and shampoos to help purify the skin. Besides these benefits, lavender is also known to have many medicinal benefits associated with it. For instance, the lavender oil is believed to have antiseptic and anti-inflammatory properties. These properties make it possible for the lavender oil to be used to heal minor burns and bug bites. More so, some studies have also shown that the consumption of lavender as tea can aid digestive complications such as vomiting, intestinal gas, upset stomach, abdominal swelling and nausea. Lavender may also be useful in treating anxiety, insomnia, depression, headaches, sores and restlessness.

15. **Thyme:** is a popular medicinal herbal plant used in cooking. Thymol is found in thyme and is popularly found in mouthwash and vapour rubs. Thymol is the substance that gives thyme its antifungal and antibacterial properties. These antifungal properties in thyme help prevent food borne diseases because it contains compounds that can decontaminate food and prevent infections in the body. Thyme has the following health benefits: aids the immune system, prevents infections from getting into the body, improves blood circulation, treats respiratory problems and soothes sore throats and coughs. Thyme can either be sprinkled as a garnish for meals, prepared as tea from its fresh leaves or applied topically as a cream.

16. **St. John's Wort:** is a medicinal herbal plant known as the most natural and traditional way to relieve symptoms of depression. This medicinal herbal plant is used to treat anxiety, mood swings, and symptoms of obsessive-compulsive disorder and feelings of withdrawal. St. John's Wort is mostly consumed as a concentrated pill or applied topically as a cream or

ointment. Significant health benefits of this medicinal herbal plant are soothing skin irritation, reduction of inflammation, aids relief from symptoms of depression and relieves anxiety and helps manage mood. St. John's Wort's fresh flowers can also be brewed for tea.

17. **Peppermint:** is a fresh medicinal herbal plant that we taste in gums, toothpastes and desserts. Peppermint is best served as tea and helps relieve tummy aches, nausea and muscle pain. More so, peppermint served as tea is a great choice for pregnant women who suffer from occasional morning sicknesses. Other health benefits of peppermint include relieves allergies, soothes muscle pain, relieves headache, reduces intestinal gas and indigestion, supports digestive health, treats bad breath, and fights bacteria. Peppermint is either taken as tea, applied topically as essential oil or inhaled as essential oil.

18. **Sage:** is a medicinal herbal plant known for its ability to support memory and fight degenerative diseases. Besides this benefit, sage is also renowned for managing diabetes with its natural compounds that have the ability to lower glucose levels. Also, the plant is commonly found on the ingredient label of several dishes and beauty products, hence the benefits are immense. Other benefits of sage includes support for the body's digestive health, rich in antioxidants, improves skin health, improves and enhances brain function, and strengthens the immune system. Sage can be used in several forms such as fresh leaves brewed for tea, sprinkled as a garnish for dishes, inhaled as an essential oil or applied topically as an essential oil.

19. **Dandelion:** is a non-edible medicinal herbal plant filed with vitamin K, vitamin C, iron, calcium and many more vitamins and minerals that are great for you. These vitamins and minerals help the body build strong bones and helps the liver stay healthy. Every part of a dandelion is good and useful for you. For instance, the

dandelion leaves are used as garnishes for several dishes, the dandelion roots are commonly used for tea, and the dandelion sap is great for your skin. Other benefits of a dandelion are detoxification of the liver and overall support for the liver health, treatment for skin infection, support overall bone health and help the body fight urinary infections. Dandelion can be consumed as tea, a garnish for several dishes or consumed as a pill.

CONCLUSION

This is the end of the book, and I must commend you, not only for starting this process of learning with me but also for making sure that you see it to the end. However, I must state that it is one thing to learn about a thing; it is an entirely different ballgame to put such knowledge into practice. You must have gained one thing from this book; however, that's not enough – you must also put the knowledge into practice in your day-to-day life. As I have stated earlier in the book, the electric food diet is a lifestyle. It is not a traditional diet that you embark upon only when you want to lose weight. The electric food diet is a diet you have to consistently follow to get your desired results and smash your diet goals. Also, remember to avoid foods with high acidity rates, which can harm the body. Instead, consume alkaline-based foods – they contain nutrients that help cleanse body organs such as kidneys, blood, and the liver. For instance, drink green tea instead of coffee, which is a caffeine product that increases the acidity level in your body. Also, packaged and processed foods are toxic; hence you avoid consuming them. Take-outs from restaurants also fall under this category. Fresh organic foods are the best for your body. They are less toxic and contain nutrients that help maintain the alkalinity level in your body. Finally, remember that we humans, you and I inclusive, are living things, hence the more we consume 'living,' organic or fresh foods, the better our body system. The more we consume 'dead' or inorganic or fortified foods, the more damage we do to our body system. I am sure this book will serve as all the boost you need to start the electric food diet, and I hope you had a great time reading the book as much as I had a great time writing it.

THANK YOU

Thank you for buying my book and I hope you enjoyed it. If you found any value in this book I would really appreciate it if you'd take a minute to post a review on Amazon about this book. I check all my reviews and love to get feedback.

This is the real reward for me knowing that I'm helping others. If you know anyone who may enjoy this book, please share the message and gift it to them.

As you work towards your goals, you may have questions or run into some issues. I'd like to be able to help you, so let's connect.
I don't charge for the assistance, so feel free to connect with me on the internet at:

Join the Smoothie Diet Lifestyle Change Facebook Group

Add Me As A Friend On Facebook

OTHER BOOKS BY AUTHOR

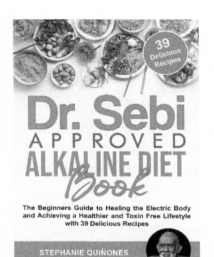

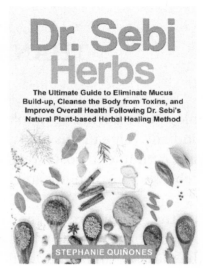

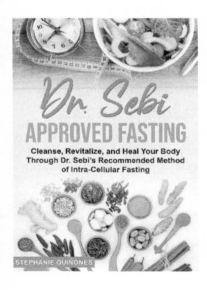

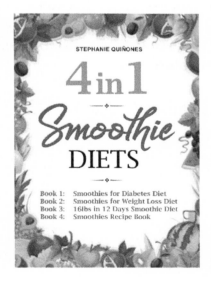

ABOUT AUTHOR

My name is Stephanie Quiñones, an entrepreneur living in the United States who loves sharing knowledge and helping others on the topic of weight-loss, healthy eating, anti-aging, and improving love life.

I'm a very passionate person who will go the extra mile and over-delivers to inspire others to lose weight, be healthy, and to achieve the sexy body they desire.

Stephanie's words of wisdom:

"I believe that knowledge is power. Everyone should improve hemselves and/or business, no matter what stage in life they're in. Whether it's to develop a better mindset or to increase profits. Moving forward is key."

Made in the USA
Monee, IL
01 November 2020

46536078R00059